Genetics of Sleep and Its Disorders

Guest Editor

ALLAN I. PACK, MBChB, PhD

SLEEP MEDICINE CLINICS

www.sleep.theclinics.com

June 2011 • Volume 6 • Number 2

SAUNDERS an imprint of ELSEVIER, Inc.

W.B. SAUNDERS COMPANY
A Division of Elsevier Inc.

1600 John F. Kennedy Boulevard • Suite 1800 • Philadelphia, PA 19103-2899

http://www.sleep.theclinics.com

SLEEP MEDICINE CLINICS Volume 6, Number 2
June 2011, ISSN 1556-407X, ISBN-13: 978-1-4557-0505-4

Editor: Sarah E. Barth
Developmental Editor: Teia Stone

Sleep Medicine Clinics (ISSN 1556-407X) is published quarterly by Elsevier Inc., 360 Park Avenue South, New York, NY 10010-1710. Months of issue are March, June, September and December. Business and Editorial Offices: 1600 John F. Kennedy Blvd., Ste. 1800, Philadelphia, PA 19103-2899. Customer Service Office: 3251 Riverport Lane, Maryland Heights, MO 63043. Periodicals postage paid at New York, NY and additional mailing offices. Subscription prices are $161.00 per year (US individuals), $80.00 (US residents), $346.00 (US institutions), $198.00 (foreign individuals), $111.00 (foreign residents), and $381.00 (foreign institutions). Foreign air speed delivery is included in all *Clinics* subscription prices. All prices are subject to change without notice. **POSTMASTER:** Send change of address to *Sleep Medicine Clinics*, Elsevier Health Sciences Division, Subscription Customer Service, 3251 Riverport Lane, Maryland Heights, MO 63043. Customer Service: **Tel: 1-800-654-2452 (U.S. and Canada); 314-447-8871 (outside U.S. and Canada). Fax: 314-447-8029. E-mail: journalscustomerservice-usa@elsevier.com (for print support); journalsonlinesupport-usa@elsevier.com (for online support).**

Reprints. For copies of 100 or more of articles in this publication, please contact the Commercial Reprints Department, Elsevier Inc., 360 Park Avenue South, New York, NY 10010-1710. Tel.: 212-633-3812; Fax: 212-462-1935; E-mail: reprints@elsevier.com.

Printed and bound by CPI Group (UK) Ltd, Croydon, CR0 4YY

Transferred to Digital Print 2011

GOAL STATEMENT

The goal of *Sleep Clinics of North America* is to keep practicing physicians up to date with current clinical practice by providing timely articles reviewing the state of the art in patient care.

ACCREDITATION

The *Sleep Clinics of North America* is planned and implemented in accordance with the Essential Areas and Policies of the Accreditation Council for Continuing Medical Education (ACCME) through the joint sponsorship of the University of Virginia School of Medicine and Elsevier. The University of Virginia School of Medicine is accredited by the ACCME to provide continuing medical education for physicians.

The University of Virginia School of Medicine designates this educational activity for a maximum of 15 *AMA PRA Category 1 Credits*™ for each issue, 60 credits per year. Physicians should only claim credit commensurate with the extent of their participation in the activity.

The American Medical Association has determined that physicians not licensed in the US who participate in this CME activity are eligible for a maximum of 15 *AMA PRA Category 1 Credits*™ for each issue, 60 credits per year.

Credit can be earned by reading the text material, taking the CME examination online at http://www.theclinics.com/home/cme, and completing the evaluation. After taking the test, you will be required to review any and all incorrect answers. Following completion of the test and evaluation, your credit will be awarded and you may print your certificate.

FACULTY DISCLOSURE/CONFLICT OF INTEREST

The University of Virginia School of Medicine, as an ACCME accredited provider, endorses and strives to comply with the Accreditation Council for Continuing Medical Education (ACCME) Standards of Commercial Support, Commonwealth of Virginia statutes, University of Virginia policies and procedures, and associated federal and private regulations and guidelines on the need for disclosure and monitoring of proprietary and financial interests that may affect the scientific integrity and balance of content delivered in continuing medical education activities under our auspices.

The University of Virginia School of Medicine requires that all CME activities accredited through this institution be developed independently and be scientifically rigorous, balanced and objective in the presentation/discussion of its content, theories and practices.

All authors/editors participating in an accredited CME activity are expected to disclose to the readers relevant financial relationships with commercial entities occurring within the past 12 months (such as grants or research support, employee, consultant, stock holder, member of speakers bureau, etc.). The University of Virginia School of Medicine will employ appropriate mechanisms to resolve potential conflicts of interest to maintain the standards of fair and balanced education to the reader. Questions about specific strategies can be directed to the Office of Continuing Medical Education, University of Virginia School of Medicine, Charlottesville, Virginia.

The faculty and staff of the University of Virginia Office of Continuing Medical Education have no financial affiliations to disclose.

The authors/editors listed below have identified no professional or financial affiliations for themselves or their spouse/partner:
Sarah Barth (Acquisitions Editor); Cynthia Brown, MD (Test Editor); Enda Byrne, PhD; Juliette Faraco, PhD; Philip R. Gehrman, PhD, CBSM; Nathan Gillespie, PhD; Namni Goel, PhD; Brian D. Kent, MB; Nicholas G. Martin, PhD; Thornton B.A. Mason II, MD, PhD, MSCE; Walter T. McNicholas, MD; David M. Raizen, MD, PhD; Silke Ryan, MD, PhD; Barbara Schormair, PhD; Keith C. Summa, BS; Nathaniel F. Watson, MD, MSc; and John E. Zimmerman, PhD.

The authors/editors listed below identified the following professional or financial affiliations for themselves or their spouse/partner:
Ann-Marie Chang, PhD's spouse is an industry funded research/investigator for Sepracor, Inc. and is a consultant for Dinsmore LLC.
Teofilo Lee-Chiong Jr, MD (Consulting Editor) is an industry funded research/investigator for Respironics and Embla.
Emmanuel Mignot, MD, PhD is a consultant for Jazz Pharmaceuticals, Actelion, Roche, Cephalon, Merck, Arena, RLS foundation, Klarman, AASM, and GSK; is on the Advisory Board of Eli Lily; paid lecture fees by Roche; an expert witness for Fred Langer, LLC; an industry sponsored reseach/investigatorfor Jazz and NIH; owns stock with Resmed and Bio Project; and has past employment with HHMI.
Allan I. Pack, MBChB, PhD (Guest Editor) receives an endowment from the Phillips/Respironics Foundation.
Fred W. Turek, PhD is an industry funded research/investigator and consultant for Servier, Merck, and Takeda; is a consultant for Astra-Zeneca; is on the Advisory Committee/Board for Philips Respironics; and is a consultant and stockholder for NuNetix, Inc.
Juliane Winklemann, MD is on the Speakers' Bureau for UCB, Vifor, Boeringer Ingelheim, and is on the Advisory Board for UCB, and field a patent to the finding in Winkelmann et al 2007.
Phyllis Zee, MD, PhD is a consultant for Merck, Sanofi Aventis, and Philips/Respironics; is on the Advisory Board for Merck, Purdue, and Philips/Respironics; and is on the Speakers' Bureau for Cephalon.

Disclosure of Discussion of Non-FDA Approved Uses for Pharmaceutical Products and/or Medical Devices.
The University of Virginia School of Medicine, as an ACCME provider, requires that all faculty presenters identify and disclose any off-label uses for pharmaceutical and medical device products. The University of Virginia School of Medicine recommends that each physician fully review all the available data on new products or procedures prior to clinical use.

TO ENROLL

To enroll in the Sleep Clinics of North America Continuing Medical Education program, call customer service at 1-800-654-2452 or visit us online at www.theclinics.com/home/cme. The CME program is available to subscribers for an additional fee of $114.00.

Sleep Medicine Clinics

THE CLINICS ARE NOW AVAILABLE ONLINE!

Access your subscription at:
www.theclinics.com

Contributors

CONSULTING EDITOR

TEOFILO LEE-CHIONG Jr, MD
Professor of Medicine and Chief, Division
of Sleep Medicine, National Jewish Health;
Associate Professor of Medicine, University
of Colorado Denver School of Medicine,
Denver, Colorado

GUEST EDITOR

ALLAN I. PACK, MBChB, PhD
John Miclot Professor of Medicine; Chief,
Division of Sleep Medicine/Department of
Medicine; Director, Center for Sleep and
Circadian Neurobiology, University of
Pennsylvania School of Medicine,
Philadelphia, Pennsylvania

AUTHORS

ENDA BYRNE, PhD
Psychiatric Genetics, Queensland Institute
of Medical Research, Brisbane, Australia

ANNE-MARIE CHANG, PhD
Instructor in Medicine, Division of Sleep
Medicine, Harvard Medical School; Associate
Neuroscientist, Department of Medicine,
Brigham and Women's Hospital, Boston,
Massachusetts

JULIETTE FARACO, PhD
Senior Research Scientist, Stanford Center
for Sleep Sciences and Medicine, Palo Alto,
California

PHILIP R. GEHRMAN, PhD, CBSM
Department of Psychiatry, University of
Pennsylvania, Philadelphia, Pennsylvania

NATHAN GILLESPIE, PhD
Department of Psychiatry, Virginia Institute for
Psychiatric and Behavior Genetics, Virginia
Commonwealth University, Richmond, Virginia

NAMNI GOEL, PhD
Assistant Professor, Division of Sleep and
Chronobiology, Unit for Experimental
Psychiatry, Department of Psychiatry,
University of Pennsylvania School of Medicine,
Philadelphia, Pennsylvania

BRIAN D. KENT, MB
Pulmonary and Sleep Disorders Unit, St.
Vincent's University Hospital, Dublin, Ireland

NICHOLAS G. MARTIN, PhD
Psychiatric Genetics, Queensland Institute
of Medical Research, Brisbane, Australia

THORNTON B.A. MASON II, MD, PhD, MSCE
Attending Physician, Division of Neurology,
The Children's Hospital of Philadelphia,
Philadelphia, Pennsylvania

WALTER T. MCNICHOLAS, MD
Director, Pulmonary and Sleep Disorders Unit,
St. Vincent's University Hospital, Dublin,
Ireland

EMMANUEL MIGNOT, MD, PhD
Craig Reynolds Professor; Director, Stanford
Center for Sleep Sciences and Medicine, Palo
Alto, California

ALLAN I. PACK, MBChB, PhD
John Miclot Professor of Medicine; Chief,
Division of Sleep Medicine/Department of
Medicine; Director, Center for Sleep and
Circadian Neurobiology, University of
Pennsylvania School of Medicine, Philadelphia,
Pennsylvania

DAVID M. RAIZEN, MD, PhD
Department of Neurology; Division of Sleep
Medicine, Department of Medicine; Center for
Sleep and Circadian Neurobiology, University
of Pennsylvania School of Medicine,
Philadelphia, Pennsylvania

SILKE RYAN, MD, PhD
Pulmonary and Sleep Disorders Unit,
St. Vincent's University Hospital, Dublin,
Ireland

BARBARA SCHORMAIR, PhD
Institute of Human Genetics, Helmholtz
Zentrum München, German Research Center
for Environmental Health, Neuherberg; Institute
of Human Genetics, Klinikum Rechts der Isar,
Technische Universität München (TUM),
Munich, Germany

KEITH C. SUMMA, BS
Center for Sleep and Circadian Biology,
Northwestern University, Evanston, Illinois

FRED W. TUREK, PhD
Charles E. and Emma H. Morrison Professor
of Biology, Department of Neurobiology and
Physiology; Director, Center for Sleep and
Circadian Biology, Northwestern University,
Evanston, Illinois

NATHANIEL F. WATSON, MD, MSc
Department of Neurology and University of
Washington Medicine Sleep Center, Seattle,
Washington

JULIANE WINKELMANN, MD
Professor of Neurogenetics, Institute of Human
Genetics, Helmholtz Zentrum München,
German Research Center for Environmental
Health, Neuherberg; Institute of Human
Genetics; Department of Neurology, Klinikum
Rechts der Isar, Technische Universität
München (TUM), Munich, Germany

PHYLLIS ZEE, MD, PhD
Professor, Department of Neurology,
Northwestern University Feinberg School
of Medicine, Chicago, Illinois

JOHN E. ZIMMERMAN, PhD
Center for Sleep and Circadian Neurobiology,
University of Pennsylvania School of Medicine,
Philadelphia, Pennsylvania

Contents

Non-mammalian Genetic Model Systems in Sleep Research   131

David M. Raizen and John E. Zimmerman

Several model systems that are amenable to genetic analysis have been added to the sleep research field in the past decade. These include the fruit fly *Drosophila melanogaster*, the round worm *Caenorhabditis elegans*, and the Zebrafish *Danio rerio*. Research in these model systems has already yielded important contributions into our understanding of the regulation and function of sleep and sleep-like states. Looking forward, these model systems hold promise to contribute for many years to the discovery of new sleep regulators, to understanding the function of genes discovered in human genetic research, and to testing hypotheses regarding the function of sleep.

The Genetics of Sleep: Insight from Rodent Models   141

Keith C. Summa and Fred W. Turek

Sleep is a fundamental behavior in higher animals that is under substantial genetic control. Genetic studies in animal models have uncovered genomic loci associated with specific traits, validated the key role of neurotransmitter systems in sleep-wake regulation, identified genes responsible for controlling sleep-wake traits, and demonstrated genetic overlap in the regulation of sleep and circadian rhythms. Future studies are expected to reveal additional genes and gene networks underlying certain sleep-wake traits, advancing understanding of the molecular basis of sleep, which may suggest answers to the question of why we sleep and provide insight into the relationship between sleep and chronic diseases.

Genetics of Electroencephalography During Wakefulness and Sleep   155

Nathaniel F. Watson

The electroencephalogram (EEG) is a readily measurable, quantifiable, heritable endophenotype of central nervous system activity in wakefulness and sleep. The EEG is the perceptible end result of synaptic neurotransmission, the basis for neuronal functioning. The EEG is well suited for studies of the genetic basis of the neurophysiology of sleep and wake. Twin and family studies have shown substantial heritability to numerous EEG phenotypes, and animal studies provide evidence that single genes may be found for quantitative EEG variants in humans. Genomic technologies are beginning to be applied to the EEG in hopes of improving understanding of this complex phenotype.

Genetics of Sleep Timing, Duration, and Homeostasis in Humans   171

Namni Goel

This article reviews the genetic underpinnings of sleep timing, duration, and homeostasis in healthy adult sleepers. Phenotypic individual differences in circadian and sleep measures as well as in neurobehavioral performance have motivated recent studies using candidate gene approaches to predict baseline (fully-rested conditions) responses and responses to sleep loss (acute total and chronic partial sleep deprivation). Several important circadian and noncircadian genetic biomarkers are involved in differential vulnerability to sleep loss. The search for other potential genetic biomarkers, using candidate gene and genome-wide association approaches, will lead to effective prediction of response and use of countermeasures to sleep loss.

Circadian rhythm sleep disorders are caused by an altered relationship between the circadian timing of sleep and the 24-hour world. Symptoms include insomnia, excessive sleepiness, and difficulty sleeping and/or waking at the desired time. Jet lag and shift work sleep disorder are circadian rhythm sleep disorders that occur when the environmental entrainment cues are rapidly changed in relation to an individual's circadian timing system. Other circadian rhythm disorders (advanced sleep phase [ASP] and delayed sleep phase [DSP]), are caused by fundamental alterations in the circadian timing of sleep relative to external time cues. Studies of ASP and DSP have led to the identification of several genetic variants, mainly in known circadian genes. Further studies are needed to identify genetic susceptibility to other circadian disorders. Better understanding of the physiologic and genetic basis of circadian rhythm disorders is crucial for the development of targeted therapies to improve sleep, performance, and health.

Little is known about the contribution of genetics to the etiology and pathophysiology of insomnia. Insomnia is associated with several negative sequelae including fatigue, irritability, and impaired concentration and memory, and is a risk factor for mood, anxiety, and substance-use disorders. Given the prevalence of insomnia and its associated public health impact, advances in our understanding of the genetic underpinnings of the disorder could lead to prevention and treatment efforts that would benefit a substantial proportion of the population. This article provides an overview of the current literature on the genetics of insomnia and discusses a possible research agenda.

Restless legs syndrome (RLS) is a common sleep-related movement disorder with a significant genetic contribution as evidenced by heritability of 50% to 60%. The view of the underlying genetic architecture evolved from that of a mendelian disease with an autosomal-dominant mode of inheritance to that of a complex multifactorial disorder with both genetic and nongenetic factors contributing to the susceptibility. Family based linkage studies and population-based association studies have identified genomic loci containing causally related genes and variants. However, the actual etiologic variants and their role in RLS pathophysiology still remain to be determined.

Narcolepsy is characterized by excessive daytime sleepiness, symptoms of dissociated REM sleep (sleep paralysis, hypnagogic hallucinations), disrupted nocturnal sleep, and cataplexy (brief episodes of muscle weakness triggered by emotions). Onset of narcolepsy is most often in childhood, peaking between 10 and 25 years of age, and once established the disease is life-long. Significant strides have recently been made in understanding narcolepsy, which can now formally be considered an autoimmune disease based the identification of strong predisposing genetic variants within the HLA and T-cell receptor loci, as well as the identification of increased levels of specific autoantibodies near disease onset.

Foreword

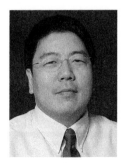

Teofilo Lee-Chiong Jr, MD
Consulting Editor

Clinicians and researchers often ignore half of the medical literature. They commonly recognize "positive" associations, such as demographics, clinical features, associated disorders, genetic linkages, and effective therapies, but often cannot explain, or are less interested in, "negative" correlations. For instance, many are aware that smoking can lead to progressive lung destruction—but why do certain smokers not develop chronic obstructive pulmonary disease? That metabolic syndrome is a major risk factor for cardiovascular events—so what protects some individuals with hyperlipidemia, glucose intolerance, and obesity from developing coronary artery disease? That exposure to specific agents, such as asbestos or polycyclic aromatic hydrocarbons, is associated with increased incidence of cancers—but are there environmental factors that reduce the likelihood of developing cancers? Why do certain therapies succeed and others fail? What genetically acquired features are responsible, in part, for healthy aging?

In the science of sleep medicine, questions such as these are just beginning to be explored, and genetics will, hopefully, provide some of the answers. Answers to questions like:

- What genes act to decrease susceptibility to obstructive sleep apnea? Why are obesity-associated phenotypes responsible for the disorder in some individuals but not others? Are there heritable ventilatory control processes that protect against upper airway obstruction and stabilize respiration during sleep? Why are nearly half of patients with obstructive sleep apnea not sleepy at all, yet others remain sleepy despite therapy with positive airway pressure?
- Why is it that Parkinson disease does not eventually develop in every person with REM sleep behavior disorder, and vice versa? Also, why does not everyone with restless legs syndrome have periodic limb movements during sleep, and vice versa? What makes a child not experience sleepwalking or night terrors when both parents did as children?
- What causes a patient with chronic insomnia to sleep better on certain evenings? Why doesn't everyone develop adjustment sleep disorder, jet lag, or shift work disorder under appropriate situations?
- Why does the severity of hypersomnia improve over time in some disorders, such as Kleine-Levin syndrome, but persist in others? What factors are responsible for patients with idiopathic hypersomnia not experiencing improvement in sleepiness following periods of sleep as patients with narcolepsy often do?
- What makes an individual less susceptible to the adverse consequences of sleep deprivation?

It has been said that children and medical students ask the most difficult questions—"Why can I see things that are behind my shadow?" or "Why do humans sleep for only eight hours each day when sleep is obviously so important for health and life?" Perhaps, it is time for sleep clinicians and researchers to start asking some difficult questions as well.

Teofilo Lee-Chiong Jr, MD
Division of Sleep Medicine
National Jewish Health
University of Colorado Denver School of Medicine
1400 Jackson Street, Room J221
Denver, CO 60206, USA

E-mail address:
Lee-ChiongT@NJC.ORG

sleep.theclinics.com

Sleep Med Clin 6 (2011) xi
doi:10.1016/j.jsmc.2011.05.001
1556-407X/11/$ – see front matter © 2011 Elsevier Inc. All rights reserved.

Preface
Genetics of Sleep and Its Disorders

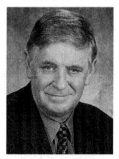

Allan I. Pack, MBChB, PhD
Guest Editor

In this issue there are reviews of many aspects of the genetics of sleep and its disorders. As the reviews point out, there are major opportunities for genetic research. Many aspects of normal sleep are heritable—sleep duration, timing of sleep, response to sleep deprivation, ECG characteristics. Moreover, many of the common sleep disorders such as insomnia, parasomnias, circadian rhythm disorders, restless legs syndrome, narcolepsy, and obstructive sleep apnea are heritable. Thus, there are many, many opportunities for genetic research. Moreover, as described throughout these reviews, there have been dramatic improvements in the technological approaches available for genotyping and continued development of these technologies.

Another major advantage for studies of the genetics of sleep and its disorders is that over the last decade, a sleep-like state has been identified in model systems, in particular, Drosophila, zebra fish, and *Caenorhabditis elegans* (for discussion of these, see Raizen and Zimmerman). This complements studies in rodent models described by Summa and Turek. Thus, sleep research is ideally positioned to first identify genes responsible for particular aspects of the phenotype in model systems and transfer findings to human studies. Identification of clock genes in Drosophila and mice with subsequent identification of variants of these genes leading to circadian rhythm disorders is a good example of this (see Chang and Zee). But the reverse is also possible, ie, identifying mutants in human studies and then assessing their functional significance by expressing these human mutations in model systems. The

recent discovery of a rare mutation in DEC2 in humans leading to short sleep is an example of this.[1] Expressing this mutation in flies and mice results in short sleep in these species.

While there are opportunities, there are also challenges. The genetic determinants of differences in the sleep phenotype and for different sleep disorders likely involve effects of many genes. Identifying these requires relatively large samples of well-phenotyped patients and controls. Currently there are no confirmed gene variants conferring risk for insomnia, parasomnias, and obstructive sleep apnea.

The two areas where progress has been made are in restless legs syndrome and narcolepsy (see Schormair and Winkelmann, and Faraco and Mignot, respectively). Using genome-wide association studies, multiple gene variants conferring risk for these disorders have been identified. There are important lessons from these examples. In restless legs syndrome, the international community developed a common phenotyping strategy based on agreed on criteria, and a questionnaire that was validated and used in studies in different countries. In narcolepsy, it was only the extreme phenotype that was studied, ie, narcolepsy with cataplexy. In studies of both disorders, there was international collaboration with cases and controls coming from different countries. This is not only true for these sleep disorders, but is also the case for the large international consortia to investigate the genetics of disorders such as diabetes, obesity, hypertension, etc. If we are to make progress in the other common sleep disorders, there is a need to develop criteria

Sleep Med Clin 6 (2011) xiii–xiv
doi:10.1016/j.jsmc.2011.04.008

that are agreed on internationally, common phenotyping strategies, and large international consortia focused on specific disorders.

Even, however, in those disorders where there has been success, much remains to be done. Genome-wide association studies (GWAS) identify common variants with small effects. Thus, not only for the sleep disorders described above but more generally in all complex genetic disorders findings from GWAS only explain a minor part of the heritability. This has directed attention to the concept that there may be rare variants in families with large effects. There could be many such variants, each with a large effect that together could explain a large part of the heritability. This concept leads to the use of new sequencing strategies, first of all exomes (protein coding regions of the genome), and then the whole genome. Studies using this approach are already starting to appear, eg, the demonstration of a rare variant of the MYH5 gene, encoding the alpha heavy chain subunit of cardiac myosin, with a high odds ratio (12.53) for sick sinus syndrome.[2] This approach will require sleep clinics to identify families with large numbers of the family having a particular sleep disorder and working collaboratively with human geneticists. It is a great opportunity for clinical/scientific collaboration.

Ultimately, this research has two major goals. First, if we can describe the genetic basis of the heritability, we should be able to use this information to identify individuals at increased risk for a disorder. (Based on data from GWAS alone, we are not close to this goal.) Second, we are likely to identify novel, as yet unknown, pathways to disease or pathways that are protective. Each such pathway becomes a therapeutic target.

In conclusion, the articles in this issue give a state-of-the-art summary of where we are with respect to knowledge about the genetics of sleep and its disorders. Our knowledge is rapidly evolving. Stay tuned.

Allan I. Pack, MBChB, PhD
Division of Sleep Medicine, Department of Medicine
Center for Sleep and Circadian Neurobiology
Translational Research Laboratories
University of Pennsylvania School of Medicine
125 South 31st Street, Suite 2100
Philadelphia, PA 19104-3403, USA

E-mail address:
pack@mail.med.upenn.edu

REFERENCES

1. He Y, Jones CR, Fujiki N, et al. The transcriptional repressor DEC2 regulates sleep length in mammals. Science 2009;325:866–70.
2. Holm H, Gudbjartsson DF, Sulem P, et al. A rare variant in MYH6 is associated with high risk of sick sinus syndrome. Nat Genet 2011;43:316–20.

Non-mammalian Genetic Model Systems in Sleep Research

David M. Raizen, MD, PhD[a,b,c,]*, John E. Zimmerman, PhD[b]

KEYWORDS

- Forward genetics • Reverse genetics • Circadian • Sleep

There are 3 principal uses of genetic model systems relevant to human sleep disorders: discovery of new genes, testing the in vivo function of gene variants associated with human sleep traits, and testing hypotheses regarding the function of sleep.

This article reviews the chief utilities of non-mammalian model system in the study of sleep. The criteria for sleep or a sleep-like state have been extensively reviewed,[1,2] as have the experiments supporting the idea that sleep is fundamentally conserved in phylogeny.[1,3–6] We will therefore start with the premise that sleep can be studied in any of the key non-mammalian model genetic systems including *D melanogaster*, *C elegans*, and *D rerio*.

GENE DISCOVERY

The oldest use of genetic model systems has been to discover genes that function in processes of interest. Such functions are often then shown to be conserved in mammalian systems. The process of finding new genes is often referred to as "forward genetics" in which one screens for a phenotype of interest following random mutagenesis of the genome. Forward genetics is hypothesis independent in that one has no a priori bias as to which genes will mutate to cause the phenotype of interest. The power of such an approach is that it can lead to novel and unexpected insights. An example of the utility of forward genetics is illustrated from genetic research in the circadian field. Nearly all components that function in the circadian clock have been discovered using forward genetics in model systems, primarily in *Drosophila*. Most of these genes have clear mammalian homologues that have also been shown to function in the mammalian clock. The clinical utility of this approach is demonstrated by Toh and colleagues[7] who have found that human families with familial advanced sleep phase syndrome (FASPS) have mutations in these same clock components.[8]

The use of forward genetics to identify noncircadian sleep regulators has been undertaken in *Drosophila*. Such screening has identified the genes *shaker* and *sleepless* as the key genes promoting sleep. *Shaker* encodes a voltage-gated potassium channel,[9] whereas *sleepless* encodes a glycosylphosphatidylinositol-anchored protein that regulates expression and function of

D.M.R. is supported by grants R01 NS064030 from the NIH and by an NARSAD Young Investigator Award, and J.E.Z. is supported by grants R21NS055821 and AG17628 from the NIH.

[a] Department of Neurology, University of Pennsylvania School of Medicine, 464 Stemmler Hall, 415 Curie Boulevard, Philadelphia, PA 19104, USA

[b] Center for Sleep and Circadian Neurobiology, University of Pennsylvania School of Medicine, Philadelphia, PA, USA

[c] Division of Sleep Medicine, Department of Medicine, University of Pennsylvania School of Medicine, Philadelphia, PA, USA

* Corresponding author. Department of Neurology, University of Pennsylvania School of Medicine, 464 Stemmler Hall, 415 Curie Boulevard, Philadelphia, PA 19104.

E-mail address: raizen@mail.med.upenn.edu

Shaker ion channels.[10,11] *Shaker* and *sleepless* mutants were the first mutants studied because of their extreme mutant phenotypes, that is, very short sleep, which facilitated their cloning and characterization. Several other short sleeping mutants have been identified among a collection of second chromosome mutants, but the molecular basis of these mutants remains unknown.[12] To date, short sleepers are the only phenotypes that have been reported in screens. Future research should include analysis of mutants with long sleep and abnormal sleep architecture.

The forward genetics approach must deal with the issue of pleiotropy and redundancy. Pleiotropy refers to the idea that more than 1 phenotype is caused by a particular genetic perturbation. A gene may be involved in the same molecular process in different cell types, it may be involved in multiple molecular processes, or the molecular process to which the gene contributes may be important for normal development in addition to adult behavior. Phenotypes that are pleiotropic may preclude analysis of sleep, which in non-mammalian species requires that the animal be able to move normally. There are several ways to address the issue of pleiotropy, including conditional activation or inactivation of a gene product to circumvent developmental lethality[13] and the use of tissue-specific RNA interference[14] or somatic recombination[15,16] to limit potentially deleterious gene expression to specific tissues. RNA interference and conditional activation can be combined to great effect to deduce the sleep function of a gene within specific tissues (see examples in **Table 1**).

Redundancy in genetic analysis refers to the idea that one or more genes have overlapping functions in the process of interest such that removing only 1 gene has no discernible phenotype. To get around redundancy, both genes functioning in a given process can be mutated. One of the strengths of using forward genetics approaches in *Drosophila* or *C elegans* from a perspective of eluding redundancy issues is that the fly and worm genomes are less duplicated than vertebrate genomes, that is, it is more likely that a single gene will fulfill a function that is fulfilled by more than 1 homologous vertebrate gene.[17,18] For example, whereas there are 3 genes encoding the protein PERIOD in mammals, there is only 1 in *Drosophila*, and whereas there are 4 genes encoding epidermal growth factor (EGF) receptors in mammals, there is only 1 in both *Drosophila* and *C elegans*.

Another approach to the issue of redundancy and pleiotropy is to overexpress rather than knock down a gene of interest. An example of this approach is illustrated by studies of the EGF signaling pathway in *C elegans*. The *C elegans* genome encodes only 1 EGF ligand, called LIN-3, and only 1 EGF receptor, called LET-23. Animals with a complete loss of function of either *lin-3* or *let-23* die because of the involvement of these gene products in signaling events controlling development. To get around this pleiotropy, Van Buskirk and Sternberg[19] overexpressed the *lin-3* gene product to induce behavioral quiescence. They then showed small but significant effects of partial loss-of-function mutations in LET-23/EGF on the natural sleep-like lethargus period.

A gene discovery approach that is driven by molecular rather than behavioral phenotypes entails the use of messenger RNA expression profiling to identify either individual genes or patterns of genes that change expression in association with behavioral state. This approach has been used to identify candidate genes that might regulate sleep. The function of these genes in regulating sleep is then tested with targeted genetic experiments. Examples of this approach include the analysis of arylalkylamine *N*-acetyltransferase,[20] the endoplasmic reticulum chaperone protein BiP,[20,21] and nuclear factor κB homologue relish.[22]

An approach that combines unbiased phenotypic analysis with gene expression studies was recently demonstrated in *Drosophila*. The approach was one of quantitative trait loci (QTL) analysis, in which the contribution of all genes in the genome can be simultaneously assessed to a quantitative phenotype of interest. The combination of phenotypic assessment of 40 wild-derived *Drosophila* lines with gene expression profiles of these lines allowed the identification of genes whose expression correlated with sleep phenotypes.[23] As in the cases mentioned earlier, the investigators then turned to a targeted approach for manipulating the function of 1 of these genes. Using this approach, they showed that mutations of each of the 3 genes— *bicoid-interacting protein 3, Tetraspanin 42Ef*, and *AKT1*—in an otherwise isogenic genetic background, conferred a sleep phenotype as predicted by the QTL analysis.

Syndecan, a transmembrane protein that regulates metabolism in the fly, was also identified in the sleep QTL analysis[23] and demonstrates a link between reduced energy metabolism and increased sleep.[24] This result obtained in *Drosophila* may be relevant to human metabolism and sleep; a minor allele in a single nucleotide polymorphism of the human homologue of the *syndecan* SDC4 is associated with higher resting energy expenditures and short sleep duration.[24]

In the fields of *C elegans* and *D rerio*, large-scale forward genetic screens for sleep phenotypes have not yet been reported. In zebra fish, an alternative to a genetic screen was recently described, in which the investigators screened a chemical library for compounds affecting sleep.[25] This novel approach led to the appreciation of novel signaling pathways regulating sleep. We anticipate that in the future, screens of chemical libraries will be applied both to *Drosophila* and *C elegans*.

IN-DEPTH CHARACTERIZATION OF GENE FUNCTION

The opposite approach to forward genetics is reverse genetics. Here, the function of a specific gene is perturbed in a very pointed hypothesis-driven way. The advantage of this approach is that one can delve into greater depths in characterizing the phenotype of the animals with the mutated gene because one has a hypothesis that predicts specific behavioral outcomes. This way, more subtle phenotypes that would not be identified in a random mutagenesis, can be uncovered. There are several examples of using model systems to study the function of specific genes in sleep regulation. Examples include the study of dopamine transporter mutants in *Drosophila*,[26] the study of ecdysone signaling in fruit flies,[27] the study of octopamine neurotransmission,[28,29] EGF signaling in both flies[30] and worms,[19] and cyclic AMP signaling in both flies[31] and worms.[32] **Table 1** summarizes the insights gained from both forward and reverse genetics approaches in non-mammalian model systems.

One of the most powerful uses of non-mammalian model organisms is in testing the in vivo significance of genes whose function in regulating sleep was first suggested based on humans genetic studies. Again, this approach was initially illustrated in the circadian field. After identification of families with FASPS bearing mutations in components of the circadian clock that were first identified in model organisms, the identified mutations were introduced into 2 model systems, the mouse and the fruit fly, to prove that the gene variants that had been identified caused the phenotype of interest (mutation of casein kinase 1 delta[8] and PER2[33]). Hence, this work is a beautiful example of coming full circle (**Fig. 1**). Genes of interest are first identified in the model organism through phenotype-driven forward genetics research; variants of these genes are then identified in humans displaying particular phenotypes of interest; and finally, these gene variants are placed back into the model system for an in-depth phenotypic characterization. As shown in **Fig. 1**, human gene variants can be identified by approaches that include genetic linkage, genome wide association studies, and whole genome sequencing.

Another recent example illustrates the power of the approach that is outlined in **Fig. 1**. Two members of a family with a naturally short sleep phenotype were found to harbor a mutation resulting in an amino acid change in DEC2, a protein which was previously characterized as a component of the circadian clock[34] but which had never been shown to affect sleep. The investigators introduced the *dec2* gene with the human variant into both mice and fruit flies to show that that variant indeed can cause a short sleep phenotype.[35] In the absence of this demonstration of causality using model organisms, it would be very difficult to prove that the variant they identified is contributing to the human sleep phenotype.

Another example of the use of non-mammalian systems in understanding genes that function in human sleep is illustrated by the work on hypocretin. Hypocretin signaling was first identified by convergent lines of work in mice[36] and dogs[37] and later shown to be central to the pathogenesis of narcolepsy.[38] But the first insight into the understanding the primordial role of hypocretin in regulating vertebrate behavioral states was gained from work in zebra fish. This system has the advantages of a simpler yet similar neuroanatomy compared with that of mammals, and with respect to the hypocretin signaling system, has the added advantage of only 1 hypocretin receptor (mammals have 2 receptors). Prober and colleagues[39] showed that overexpression of hypocretin leads to hyperactivity and reduced sleep at a time (lights off) when the animals are normally quiescent. Yokogawa and colleagues[40] showed that deletion of the single hypocretin receptor resulted in behavioral state instability during the fish's normal sleep time. This work then established an ancient role for hypocretin both in promoting arousal and in stabilizing behavioral states.

Although a potential disadvantage of zebra fish is the difficulty of performing traditional electrophysiologic recordings from live animals, a recent technological advance has made this apparent disadvantage far less of a concern.[41] These investigators expressed in hypocretinergic neurons a protein genetically engineered to emit light when bound to calcium. Because zebra fish are small and relatively transparent, light emitted by deep brain tissue can be recorded outside the animal. They were thus able to follow the physiologic activity of these neurons in awake,

Table 1
Genes identified as sleep regulators in non-mammalian model systems

Organism	Gene	Molecular Identity	Phenotype[a]	Insight Gained
Drosophila	Shaker	Pore-forming subunit of a voltage gated potassium channel	Less sleep	Membrane excitability affects sleep/wake
	Sleepless[10]	Novel GPI-anchored protein that regulates Shaker	Less sleep	Membrane excitability affects sleep/wake
	Hyperkinetic[59]	Accessory subunit of Shaker potassium channel	Less sleep	Membrane excitability affects sleep/wake
	Fumin[26]	Dopamine transporter	Less sleep and hyper-responsiveness	Dopamine promotes arousal
	EcR[27]	Ecdysone receptor	Less sleep	Steroid signaling promotes sleep
	Rutabaga[31]	Adenylate Cyclase	More sleep	cAMP signaling promotes wake
	Dunce[31]	cAMP-specific phosphodiesterase	Less sleep	cAMP signaling promotes wake
	D-CREB[31]	Cyclic AMP Response Element Binding Protein	More sleep	cAMP signaling promotes wake
	ATF-2[60]	CRE binding protein activated by stress/locomotor activity	Less sleep[b]	Activation of ATF-2 promotes sleep
	Syndecan[24]	Trans-membrane protein involved in energy metabolism	More sleep	A reduction in metabolic rate promotes sleep
	Spargel[24]	PGC-1	More sleep	A reduction in metabolic rate promotes sleep
	Rhomboid[30]	Membrane-bound protease that activates EGFR ligand	More sleep[b]	EGFR activation promotes sleep
	Resistant to dieldrin[61]	GABA$_A$ receptor	Less sleep[b]	GABA promotes sleep
	Tyrosine decarboxylase 2[28]	Enzyme that converts tyrosine to tyramine, the substrate for octopamine	More sleep	Octopamine promotes wake
	Tyramine β hydroxylase[28]	Enzyme that converts tyramine to octopamine	More sleep	Octopamine promotes wake
	5-HT$_{1A}$[62]	Serotonin receptor	Less sleep	Serotonin promotes sleep
	Fmr1[63]	RNA-binding protein	More sleep	Fmr1 promotes wake

Organism	Gene	Protein	Phenotype	Function
C elegans	pde-4[32]	cAMP-specific phosphodiesterase	Hyper-responsiveness	cAMP promotes wake
	acy-1[32]	Adenylate cyclase	Hyper-responsiveness[c]	cAMP promotes wake
	kin-2[64]	Regulatory subunit of cAMP-dependent protein kinase	Hyper-responsiveness	cAMP promotes wake
	egl-4[32]	cGMP dependent protein kinase	Hyper-responsiveness and reduced quiescence	cGMP promotes sleep
	let-23[19]	EGF receptor	Reduced quiescence	EGF signaling required for function of sleep-inducing neuron ALA
	plc-3[19]	Phospholipase C-gamma	Reduced quiescence	EGF signaling in ALA is via phospholipase C gamma.
	lin-3[19]	EGF receptor ligand	Increased quiescence[c]	EGF signaling promotes sleep
D rerio	Hypocretin[39]	—	Reduced quiescence[c]	Hypocretin promotes wake
	Hypocretin receptor[40]	—	Fragmented nocturnal sleep	Hypocretin signaling is required for behavioral state stability

Abbreviations: ATF-2, activating transcription factor-2; cAMP, cyclic AMP; cGMP, cyclic GMP; CRE, cAMP response element; CREB, CRE-binding protein; EGF, epidermal growth factor; EGFR, epidermal growth factor receptor; GABA, γ-aminobutyric acid; GPI, glycosylphosphatidylinositol; 5-HT$_{1A}$, 5-hydroxytryptamine receptor.

[a] Unless otherwise indicated, phenotype is that of a reduction in gene function.

[b] Based on RNA interference knockout.

[c] Based on analysis of gain-of-function phenotype.

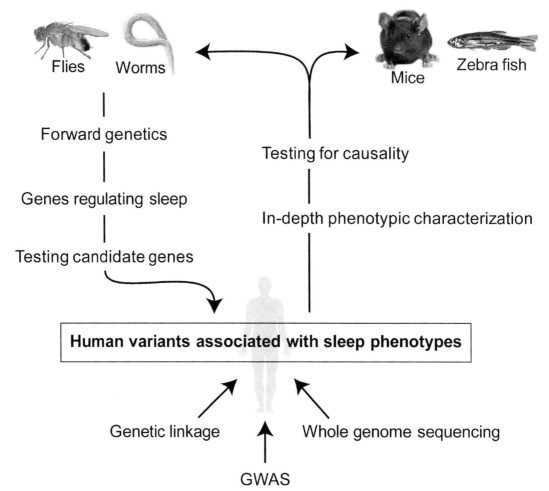

Fig. 1. Scheme for using genetic model systems to study genes involved in human sleep disorders. GWAS, genome wide association studies.

unrestrained, behaving animals. This method, which can be used to monitor the activity of any neuron cell group for which there is a specific promoter, has the advantage over traditional electrophysiology in being noninvasive and allowing simultaneous monitoring of all cells in a functional group. The same method has been used in *Drosophila*,[42] although it has not yet been used for the study of sleep.

TESTING FUNCTIONS OF SLEEP

Recent years have witnessed an increasing appreciation of the effects of acute total sleep deprivation and of chronic partial sleep restriction on human disease. The question of the function of sleep is therefore no longer purely an academic one and has tremendous implications both to public policy, particularly in the occupational health arena, and to possible therapeutic interventions to prevent or slow disease. Research in simple non-mammalian animal models may allow for testing specific hypotheses regarding the function of sleep.

Among the many theories regarding the function of sleep, 2 have stood out in recent years: (1) sleep as a restorative state for brain energetics and (2) sleep as a state promoting nervous system plasticity. The idea that sleep is restorative to brain metabolic storage pools has been tested in *Drosophila*, in which glycogen levels fluctuate in the brain but not in the body in a circadian manner.[43] Glycogen stores measured in whole animals (brains and bodies) correlate with sleep amounts in male flies,[44] and brain glycogen stores decrease after 3 hours of acute sleep deprivation.[43] In contrast to the response of brain glycogen levels to acute sleep deprivation, the whole body glycogen level is reduced by repetitive mechanical stimulation, regardless of whether the stimulation is applied during the wake or sleep period. The ability to study mutants in *Drosophila* allows one to get past correlation and to test causal relationships between energy stores and sleep or sleep homeostasis.[44,45]

With respect to synaptic plasticity, this theory has its roots in the observation of increased sleep and sleep pressure during the development of animals. With rare exceptions,[46] maximal rest or sleep occurs at birth, with the amount gradually decreasing as animals grow to the adult stage. This fact is true not only for terrestrial mammals but also for zebra fish, which show longer quiescent bouts as larvae[39,40]; fruit flies, whose sleep amounts decline as they age[20,47]; and round worms, which show long periods of behavioral quiescence predominantly during the larval stages.[32] Alternative specific hypotheses regarding the cellular mechanisms of brain plasticity have been proposed.[48,49] Both these alternative theories propose that changes in synaptic strength occur as a function of behavioral state, although in one case, the change is predominantly in the positive direction (ie, synapses are potentiated), whereas in the other, changes are in the negative direction (ie, synapses are depressed).

Work in model genetic organisms has provided some illumination into these theories. Circadian changes in *Drosophila* neuronal terminals have been observed.[50,51] Gilestro and colleagues[52] showed that independent from circadian effects, sleep results in reduced expression of both presynaptic and postsynaptic proteins. Donlea and colleagues[53] showed that sleep deprivation results in an increase in synaptic terminals of *Drosophila* lateral neurons, again suggesting that wake and sleep promote synaptic growth and depression, respectively. Applebaum and colleagues[54] exploited zebra fish's transparency to study the dynamics of synaptic structure in specific neurons as a function of the circadian time and behavioral state. They observed a clear reduction in synapses during the nighttime relative to the daytime. Sleep deprivation had only a modest effect on synapses, suggesting that at least in the zebra fish hypocretinergic synapses that they studied, the predominant inputs to synaptic change are circadian and not sleep/wake cycles.

The *C elegans* sleep-like state lethargus period occurs not on a circadian time frame but rather on a developmental time frame. However, analogous to the circadian system, cycling of expression of the worm orthologues of PERIOD protein is observed to occur with larval cycles.[55] With respect to the total number of cells and to the size of its nervous system, *C elegans* is the simplest animal to date for which a sleep or a sleep-like state has been described. Understanding the events that occur during the lethargus period may therefore give clues as to the core function of sleep. Studies in this respect are ongoing, but a few preliminary comments can be made. First, as has been proposed, the observation of sleep-like behavior predominantly during development and not in the adult worm suggests a role for this behavior in development.[56] Second, over one-fourth of the 302 neurons in the *C elegans* adult nervous system is born during larval development. These neurons must get incorporated into the existing circuitry, necessitating the formation of new synapses as well as the elimination of some old synapses. Thus, *C elegans* is an excellent model system for the study of nervous system plasticity and its relationship to sleep-like states. Third, lethargus marks the time in which the animal completes the synthesis and assembly of a new cuticle and escapes from the old cuticle. Molting is a process that is executed primarily by epithelial cells. Hence, there is a clear relationship of *C elegans* sleep-like state to events that occur outside the nervous system. This observation leads to reconsideration of the dogma that sleep serves a function unique to the nervous system.[57] Finally, the association with the molt, which is presumably a biosynthetically active process in the worm, is in keeping with theories suggesting that sleep and sleep-like state are associated with anabolic cellular processes.[58]

SUMMARY

With the explosion in the number of genome wide association studies and the anticipated frequent use of whole genome sequencing to identify human gene variants associated with disease, it has become increasingly important to identify the proper approach for testing the in vivo significance of identified variants. Model genetic systems including mice, fruit flies, round worms, and zebra fish allow one to perform such testing. *C elegans* and *Drosophila* offer the additional advantages of rapidity of experiments and their use in the identification of new sleep regulating genes, variations in which may also affect human sleep.

ACKNOWLEDGMENTS

We thank Jennifer Montoya for assistance in manuscript preparation.

REFERENCES

1. Zimmerman JE, Raizen DM, Pack AI. Conservation of sleep: insights from non-mammalian model systems. Trends Neurosci 2008;31:371–6.

2. Hendricks JC, Sehgal A, Pack AI. The need for a simple animal model to understand sleep. Prog Neurobiol 2000;61:339–51.

3. Cirelli C, Tononi G. Is sleep essential? PLoS Biol 2008;6:e216.

4. Allada R, Siegel JM. Unearthing the phylogenetic roots of sleep. Curr Biol 2008;18:R670–9.

5. Cirelli C. The genetic and molecular regulation of sleep: from fruit flies to humans. Nat Rev Neurosci 2009;10:549–60.

6. Cirelli C, Bushey D. Sleep and wakefulness in Drosophila melanogaster. Ann N Y Acad Sci 2008; 1129:323–9.

7. Toh KL, Jones CR, He Y, et al. An hPer2 phosphory-lation site mutation in familial advanced sleep phase syndrome. Science 2001;291:1040–3.

8. Xu Y, Padiath QS, Shapiro RE, et al. Functional consequences of a CKIdelta mutation causing familial advanced sleep phase syndrome. Nature 2005;434:640–4.

9. Cirelli C, Bushey D, Hill S, et al. Reduced sleep in Drosophila Shaker mutants. Nature 2005;434: 1087–92.

10. Koh K, Joiner WJ, Wu MN, et al. Identification of SLEEPLESS, a sleep-promoting factor. Science 2008;321:372–6.

11. Wu MN, Joiner WJ, Dean T, et al. SLEEPLESS, a Ly-6/neurotoxin family member, regulates the levels, localization and activity of Shaker. Nat Neurosci 2010;13:69–75.

12. Wu MN, Koh K, Yue Z, et al. A genetic screen for sleep and circadian mutants reveals mechanisms underlying regulation of sleep in Drosophila. Sleep 2008;31:465–72.

13. Elliott DA, Brand AH. The GAL4 system: a versatile system for the expression of genes. Methods Mol Biol 2008;420:79–95.

14. Perrimon N, Ni JQ, Perkins L. In vivo RNAi: today and tomorrow. Cold Spring Harb Perspect Biol 2010;2:a003640.

15. Evans CJ, Olson JM, Ngo KT, et al. G-TRACE: rapid Gal4-based cell lineage analysis in Drosophila. Nat Methods 2009;6:603–5.

16. Griffin R, Sustar A, Bonvin M, et al. The twin spot generator for differential Drosophila lineage analysis. Nat Methods 2009;6:600–2.

17. Gu Z, Cavalcanti A, Chen FC, et al. Extent of gene duplication in the genomes of Drosophila, nematode, and yeast. Mol Biol Evol 2002;19:256–62.

18. Pebusque MJ, Coulier F, Birnbaum D, et al. Ancient large-scale genome duplications: phylogenetic and linkage analyses shed light on chordate genome evolution. Mol Biol Evol 1998;15:1145–59.

19. Van Buskirk C, Sternberg PW. Epidermal growth factor signaling induces behavioral quiescence in Caenorhabditis elegans. Nat Neurosci 2007;10:1300–7.

20. Shaw PJ, Cirelli C, Greenspan RJ, et al. Correlates of sleep and waking in Drosophila melanogaster. Science 2000;287:1834–7.

21. Naidoo N, Casiano V, Cater J, et al. A role for the molecular chaperone protein BiP/GRP78 in Drosophila sleep homeostasis. Sleep 2007;30: 557–65.

22. Williams JA, Sathyanarayanan S, Hendricks JC, et al. Interaction between sleep and the immune response in Drosophila: a role for the NFkappaB relish. Sleep 2007;30:389–400.

23. Harbison ST, Carbone MA, Ayroles JF, et al. Co-regulated transcriptional networks contribute to natural genetic variation in Drosophila sleep. Nat Genet 2009;41:371–5.

24. De Luca M, Klimentidis YC, Casazza K, et al. A conserved role for syndecan family members in the regulation of whole-body energy metabolism. PLoS One 2010;5:e11286.

25. Rihel J, Prober DA, Arvanites A, et al. Zebrafish behavioral profiling links drugs to biological targets and rest/wake regulation. Science 2010; 327:348–51.

26. Kume K, Kume S, Park SK, et al. Dopamine is a regulator of arousal in the fruit fly. J Neurosci 2005;25: 7377–84.

27. Ishimoto H, Kitamoto T. The steroid molting hormone Ecdysone regulates sleep in adult Drosophila melanogaster. Genetics 2010;185:269–81.

28. Crocker A, Sehgal A. Octopamine regulates sleep in drosophila through protein kinase A-dependent mechanisms. J Neurosci 2008;28:9377–85.

29. Crocker A, Shahidullah M, Levitan IB, et al. Identification of a neural circuit that underlies the effects of octopamine on sleep:wake behavior. Neuron 2010;65:670–81.

30. Foltenyi K, Greenspan RJ, Newport JW. Activation of EGFR and ERK by rhomboid signaling regulates the consolidation and maintenance of sleep in Drosophila. Nat Neurosci 2007;10:1160–7.

31. Hendricks JC, Williams JA, Panckeri K, et al. A non-circadian role for cAMP signaling and CREB activity in Drosophila rest homeostasis. Nat Neurosci 2001; 4:1108–15.

32. Raizen DM, Zimmerman JE, Ta UD, et al. Lethargus is a C. elegans sleep like state. Nature 2008;451: 569–72.

33. Xu Y, Toh KL, Jones CR, et al. Modeling of a human circadian mutation yields insights into clock regulation by PER2. Cell 2007;128:59–70.

34. Honma S, Kawamoto T, Takagi Y, et al. Dec1 and Dec2 are regulators of the mammalian molecular clock. Nature 2002;419:841–4.

35. He Y, Jones CR, Fujiki N, et al. The transcriptional repressor DEC2 regulates sleep length in mammals. Science 2009;325:866–70.

36. Chemelli RM, Willie JT, Sinton CM, et al. Narcolepsy in orexin knockout mice: molecular genetics of sleep regulation. Cell 1999;98:437–51.

37. Lin L, Faraco J, Li R, et al. The sleep disorder canine narcolepsy is caused by a mutation in the hypocretin (orexin) receptor 2 gene. Cell 1999;98:365–76.

38. Siegel JM. Hypocretin (orexin): role in normal behavior and neuropathology. Annu Rev Psychol 2004;55:125–48.

39. Prober DA, Rihel J, Onah AA, et al. Hypocretin/orexin overexpression induces an insomnia-like phenotype in zebrafish. J Neurosci 2006;26:13400–10.

40. Yokogawa T, Marin W, Faraco J, et al. Characterization of sleep in zebrafish and insomnia in hypocretin receptor mutants. PLoS Biol 2007;5:2379–97.

41. Naumann EA, Kampff AR, Prober DA, et al. Monitoring neural activity with bioluminescence during natural behavior. Nat Neurosci 2010;13:513–20.

42. Martin JR, Rogers KL, Chagneau C, et al. In vivo bioluminescence imaging of Ca signalling in the brain of Drosophila. PLoS One 2007;2:e275.

43. Zimmerman JE, Mackiewicz M, Galante RJ, et al. Glycogen in the brain of Drosophila melanogaster: diurnal rhythm and the effect of rest deprivation. J Neurochem 2004;88:32–40.

44. Harbison ST, Sehgal A. Quantitative genetic analysis of sleep in Drosophila melanogaster. Genetics 2008; 178:2341–60.

45. Thimgan MS, Suzuki Y, Seugnet L, et al. The perilipin homologue, lipid storage droplet 2, regulates sleep homeostasis and prevents learning impairments following sleep loss. PLoS Biol 2010;8:e1000466.

46. Lyamin O, Pryaslova J, Lance V, et al. Animal behaviour: continuous activity in cetaceans after birth. Nature 2005;435:1177.

47. Koh K, Evans JM, Hendricks JC, et al. A Drosophila model for age-associated changes in sleep:wake cycles. Proc Natl Acad Sci U S A 2006;103: 13843–7.

48. Tononi G, Cirelli C. Sleep and synaptic homeostasis: a hypothesis. Brain Res Bull 2003;62:143–50.

49. Aton SJ, Seibt J, Dumoulin M, et al. Mechanisms of sleep-dependent consolidation of cortical plasticity. Neuron 2009;61:454–66.

50. Mehnert KI, Beramendi A, Elghazali F, et al. Circadian changes in Drosophila motor terminals. Dev Neurobiol 2007;67:415–21.

51. Fernandez MP, Berni J, Ceriani MF. Circadian remodeling of neuronal circuits involved in rhythmic behavior. PLoS Biol 2008;6:e69.

52. Gilestro GF, Tononi G, Cirelli C. Widespread changes in synaptic markers as a function of sleep and wakefulness in Drosophila. Science 2009;324: 109–12.

53. Donlea JM, Ramanan N, Shaw PJ. Use-dependent plasticity in clock neurons regulates sleep need in Drosophila. Science 2009;324:105–8.

54. Appelbaum L, Wang G, Yokogawa T, et al. Circadian and homeostatic regulation of structural synaptic plasticity in hypocretin neurons. Neuron 2010;68: 87–98.

55. Jeon M, Gardner HF, Miller EA, et al. Similarity of the C. elegans developmental timing protein LIN-42 to circadian rhythm proteins. Science 1999;286:1141–6.

56. Roffwarg HP, Muzio JN, Dement WC. Ontogenetic development of the human sleep-dream cycle. Science 1966;152:604–19.

57. Hobson JA. Sleep is of the brain, by the brain and for the brain. Nature 2005;437:1254–6.

58. Mackiewicz M, Shockley KR, Romer MA, et al. Macromolecule biosynthesis: a key function of sleep. Physiol Genomics 2007;31:441–57.

59. Bushey D, Huber R, Tononi G, et al. Drosophila Hyperkinetic mutants have reduced sleep and impaired memory. J Neurosci 2007;27:5384–93.

60. Shimizu H, Shimoda M, Yamaguchi T, et al. Drosophila ATF-2 regulates sleep and locomotor activity in pacemaker neurons. Mol Cell Biol 2008; 28:6278–89.

61. Agosto J, Choi JC, Parisky KM, et al. Modulation of GABAA receptor desensitization uncouples sleep onset and maintenance in Drosophila. Nat Neurosci 2008;11:354–9.

62. Yuan Q, Joiner WJ, Sehgal A. A sleep-promoting role for the Drosophila serotonin receptor 1A. Curr Biol 2006;16:1051–62.

63. Bushey D, Tononi G, Cirelli C. The Drosophila fragile X mental retardation gene regulates sleep need. J Neurosci 2009;29:1948–61.

64. van der Linden AM, Wiener S, You YJ, et al. The EGL-4 PKG acts with KIN-29 salt-inducible kinase and protein kinase A to regulate chemoreceptor gene expression and sensory behaviors in Caenorhabditis elegans. Genetics 2008;180:1475–91.

The Genetics of Sleep: Insight from Rodent Models

Keith C. Summa, BS[a], Fred W. Turek, PhD[a,b,*]

KEYWORDS

• Sleep • Genetics • Animal models • Rodents
• Circadian rhythms

Substantial evidence demonstrates that many sleep-wake traits as well as several sleep disorders are under significant genetic control in organisms as diverse as flies, rodents, and humans. Perhaps the most convincing evidence comes from twin studies in humans, where, in addition to overall gross central nervous system (CNS) architecture and regional electrical activity patterns, complex electroencephalogram (EEG) traits exhibit a much higher concordance in monozygotic twins than in dizygotic twins.[1–3] The EEG patterns in twins nearly match those recorded in the same individual on different occasions,[4] highlighting the crucial role of genes in regulating complex EEG traits. Additionally, specific sleep traits, such as the total amount or timing of sleep, are also under significant genetic control: it has been estimated that approximately 50% of the variance of these traits is due to genetic factors[5] (see the article by Namni Goel elsewhere in this issue).

These convincing data in humans are complemented by extensive work in rodents. Pioneering studies undertaken by Valatx and colleagues[6–8] documented the segregation of sleep traits, mainly those related to rapid eye movement (REM) sleep, in inbred, recombinant-inbred (RI), and hybrid mice. Although the underlying role of genetics in the regulation of sleep-wake traits has been appreciated for decades, only recently have individual genes begun to be identified, beginning with the hypocretin-2 receptor gene, which was shown in 1999 to be mutated in canine narcolepsy.[9] The number of identified genes remains low, and the precise molecular basis of the function of these genes in sleep-wake regulation is unknown. The complexity and range of phenotypes underlying mammalian sleep suggest that many genes as well as complex networks of interacting genes working in unison are integrated in the endogenous control of sleep and the converse state, wake. The substantial phenotypic variability of specific sleep traits and the relatively significant influence of environmental factors on sleep-wake parameters have made the identification of specific genes difficult. In spite of these difficulties, technologic advances in genomic sequencing, mapping, and analysis, in combination with high-throughput sleep screening, offer great promise for the identification of the specific genetic components underlying sleep-wake traits in the near future. Additionally, sophisticated systems biology approaches can be integrated into these analyses in a powerful manner to

This work was supported by Grant Nos. P01 AG114212 and T32 HL007909 from the National Institutes of Health.

The authors have nothing to disclose.

[a] Center for Sleep and Circadian Biology, Northwestern University, 2205 Tech Drive, Evanston, IL 60208-3520, USA

[b] Department of Neurobiology and Physiology, Northwestern University, 2205 Tech Drive, Evanston, IL 60208-3520, USA

* Corresponding author. Center for Sleep and Circadian Biology, Northwestern University, 2205 Tech Drive, Evanston, IL 60208-3520.

E-mail address: fturek@northwestern.edu

uncover how interacting genetic networks contribute to the regulation of certain aspects of sleep. Together, these approaches offer tremendous potential for sleep researchers and are expected to further understanding of which genes are involved in regulating sleep and how these genes work together to form the molecular basis of the complex behavior of sleep.

This article summarizes the literature addressing the genetic basis of sleep in rodents, in particular mice. It begins by describing studies exploring gene expression during wake and sleep as well as in response to sleep deprivation. Then several comprehensive studies undertaken to identify genomic loci and candidate genes that regulate quantitative sleep traits in segregating mouse populations are reviewed, including novel attempts to test the hypothesis that the regulation of gene expression underlies particular traits. Next, studies using mutagenesis, transgenic, and knockout technologies in the mouse to address the role of individual genes in sleep are highlighted, with special emphasis on genes controlling circadian rhythms, including the sleep-wake rhythm. How these studies in mice indicate that the genetic control of sleep is highly integrated with the genetic regulation of circadian rhythms is discussed. Recent analyses of sleep in flies have demonstrated the validity of this invertebrate organism as a valid model system and have contributed to understanding of the genetic regulation of sleep, but discussion of this topic is beyond the scope of this review (see Refs.[10–12] and article by Raizen and Zimmerman elsewhere in this issue).

Both sleep and circadian rhythms are highly conserved, crucial physiologic processes. Therefore, disruptions of sleep or circadian rhythms (or both) are expected to have significant detrimental effects on an organism. A rapidly growing body of epidemiologic and experimental evidence now demonstrates that sleep-wake and/or circadian rhythm disturbances are linked to a range of chronic diseases, both central (eg, psychiatric and neurodegenerative disease[13]) and peripheral (eg, metabolic and cardiovascular disease[14–16]) that have profound medical, public health, and economic costs in humans. Thus, animal models demonstrating that sleep and circadian rhythms are regulated, to some extent, in unison at the genetic level serve as important experimental tools necessary to uncover the mechanisms linking the genetic control of sleep and circadian rhythms to disease pathophysiology. These are expected to provide insight into the underlying basis of the widespread epidemiologic and experimental observations associating sleep-wake and circadian disturbances with disease in humans.

ANALYSIS OF GENE EXPRESSION ACROSS SLEEP AND WAKE AS WELL AS AFTER SLEEP DEPRIVATION

Initial studies examining variation in gene expression across sleep and wake states identified activation of rapid response genes, also known as immediate early genes (IEGs), including *Fos*, during wake compared with sleep.[17–19] Most IEGs, which are expressed in activated neurons, encode transcription factors that may lie upstream of critical signaling cascades. Thus, IEGs can be used to identify neuroanatomic regions activated by changes in arousal state. For example, although the majority of the cortex is active with higher levels of IEG expression during wake, there is a small group of γ-aminobutyric acid-ergic (GABAergic) neurons also expressing neuronal nitric oxide synthase that exhibit increased *Fos* expression during non-REM (NREM) sleep.[20] This set of sleep-active neurons may represent a cortical region important in regulating firing patterns necessary during NREM sleep, namely the synchronous firing underlying EEG delta power (slow wave activity).[21]

Similarly, *Fos* expression is higher during sleep in the ventrolateral preoptic area,[22] a hypothalamic region with extensive inhibitory GABAergic projections to wake-promoting centers,[23] suggesting a critical role in the regulation of arousal and wake. The neuroanatomic studies of the ventrolateral preoptic area as well as several other hypothalamic nuclei formed the basis of a model proposing hypothalamic regulation of sleep via a switch mediating alternating activity of arousal-promoting and sleep-promoting nuclei.[24]

Although these studies of IEG and *Fos* expression have contributed significant advances to understanding of the neuroanatomic and physiologic regulation of sleep, they have not provided clear insight into the genetic control of sleep. The expression patterns do not allow differentiating between genes controlling sleep-state changes and/or patterns of neuronal activation as opposed to those merely responding to them. One possibility may be that expression differences between wake and sleep are indicative of compartmentalization of cellular functions to specific behavioral states, for example, transcriptional activity, as directed by the IEGs, may be performed preferentially during wake whereas protein synthesis may predominate during sleep. This hypothesis has some support from earlier studies finding a correlation between the amount of slow wave sleep and incorporation of the radiolabeled amino acid leucine into protein in the brain[25,26]; however, the data on protein dynamics related to sleep are limited. Thus, although analysis of differential gene expression across sleep and wake states raises hypotheses about potential cellular functions during these states, it does not generate clear conclusions regarding the genetic regulation of sleep-state transitions or sleep-wake traits in general.

More recent studies of gene expression have used microarrays to perform comprehensive, unbiased analyses of global expression patterns across sleep and wake, often of thousands of expressed transcripts in a single brain region. The first such large-scale study compared transcripts collected from both undisturbed (and presumably sleeping) and sleep-deprived rats at 6:00 PM as well as from undisturbed rats at 6:00 AM that were awake most of the night.[27] Approximately 10% of the more than 15,000 transcripts detected in the cerebral cortex varied across day and night, and approximately half of these (corresponding to approximately 5% of the total) differed between sleep and wake regardless of the time of day, indicating that many genes respond directly to sleep-wake cycles. Similar results were obtained in the cerebellum, a region not typically associated with sleep, suggesting that perhaps all neurons require cycles of rest and activity, although describing sleep at the level of single cells is premature and speculative at best.[21]

Analyses of individual transcripts differentially regulated across sleep-wake states indicate that certain categories of genes tend to be increased during wake or sleep. The mRNAs up-regulated during wake include, but are not limited to, those involved in energy-related processes (eg, mitochondrial genes implicated in oxidative phosphorylation), transcriptional regulation, circadian rhythms, responses to stress, glutamatergic neurotransmission, and long-term potentiation.[27] Those transcripts increased during sleep relative to wake include categories such as translational regulation, membrane trafficking, membrane potential, and synaptic plasticity.[27] These results suggest that several broad classes of genes and expressed transcripts may be associated with or dependent on particular sleep-wake states, but again they do not provide clear insight into the genes underlying specific sleep-wake traits themselves.

Other microarray studies have explored patterns of gene expression across the entire day in both sleeping and sleep-deprived mice. One study found that many transcripts involved in biosynthetic processes and molecular transport were up-regulated during sleep, a pattern particularly evident in genes for cholesterol synthesis and lipid transport.[28] This observation is broadly consistent with the intuitive hypothesis that sleep is restorative at the molecular and/or cellular level within the CNS, although the precise details are unknown and, at present, convincing experimental support for this hypothesis is lacking.

Another large-scale study that included 3 different inbred strains of mice compared expression in sleep-deprived versus control animals every 4 hours throughout the 24-hour day.[29] The majority of rhythmic transcripts in the brain (approximately 1600 of just over 2000) did not continue to cycle with sleep deprivation, suggesting that many diurnal patterns of gene expression may be dependent on sleep-wake state as opposed to direct circadian factors. Also, many of these rhythmic transcripts were strain-specific. Therefore, analysis of the relatively few transcripts that cycled in a consistent manner across each of these strains is expected to highlight genes that are most functionally relevant for basic sleep processes. *Homer1a* (a truncated form of *Homer1*), a gene implicated in glutamate neurotransmission and believed important for cellular calcium homeostasis,[30] demonstrated the most consistent changes across species. This gene is located in a region of the genome that has been demonstrated to regulate, in part, the recovery from sleep deprivation (discussed later).[31]

Although these studies reveal data regarding transcriptional changes associated with sleep states, there are several limitations to consider. First, many of the observed changes may be species-specific or strain-specific and may be unique to the particular experimental conditions of each study. Second, it is impossible to determine directionality, namely whether these transcripts cause or simply respond to sleep state changes. Furthermore, sleep state changes may require only subtle alterations in expression levels that cannot be detected using conventional microarray approaches, although new sequence technologies, such as RNA-seq,[32] may partially address this limitation. In addition, although longer effects are possible, transcriptional regulation is expected to exert effects mainly on a time scale of minutes to hours whereas sleep state changes have the ability to occur over shorter periods of time. Therefore, there may be physiologic processes that alter or affect neuronal function over a span of seconds, which may directly and rapidly regulate sleep state changes independent of differences in gene expression. For example, posttranslational modification of proteins may underlie rapid alterations in protein function necessary for sleep state changes. Unfortunately, protein changes such as these are difficult to measure in vivo in a high-throughput fashion in large numbers of animals, precluding comprehensive studies exploring how protein modifications are related to sleep states at this time.

Another consideration is that studies including the measurement of gene expression during or after sleep deprivation require physical manipulation of the animals to maintain wakefulness. This intervention may itself induce changes in gene expression that are different from endogenous changes regulating natural sleep in an undisturbed environment (or sleep in humans). In spite of these potential limitations, the observation that a significant portion of mRNAs (approximately 5%) varies across sleep and wake indicates that sleep and transcription are linked. These data can be integrated with neuroanatomic and physiologic information to determine the functional significance of the changes in expression and how they may relate to the regulation of sleep-wake physiology as well as to the general functions of sleep.

IDENTIFICATION OF GENETIC LOCI CONTROLLING SLEEP-WAKE TRAITS

One approach (described previously) uses dynamic gene expression data across sleep-wake states and in response to sleep deprivation in an attempt to determine how global transcription alterations are associated with sleep state changes. An alternative approach exploits natural phenotypic variation among inbred strains of mice to determine which regions of the genome are responsible for the variation and, therefore, regulation of particular traits that differ between distinct strains. In this approach, two parental strains that vary with respect to the trait of interest are crossed, and their progeny (F1) are then intercrossed to create second-generation offspring (F2), containing individuals that are mosaics of genetic material from each parental strain. Careful analysis of these F2 animals is expected to reveal the mode of inheritance of the trait of interest, which will be complex for behavioral phenotypes, such as sleep. Genomic sequence analysis of these F2 offspring using polymorphic markers different between the two parental strains then allows mapping of chromosomal regions associated with the trait of interest. The underlying assumption is that genetic markers that are physically linked to the genes underlying the trait of interest segregate with the trait. This approach has been especially successful for monogenic traits inherited in predicted mendelian probabilities, and it has also become increasingly amenable for application to the study of complex traits arising from a combination of environmental factors and several genetic loci of relatively smaller effect sizes.[33]

This approach, termed, *quantitative trait loci (QTL) analysis*, is a powerful tool to uncover the genomic basis for phenotypic traits. A major weakness of this approach, however, regards the difficulty in identifying particular genes affecting the trait once the relevant genomic region is known. Often, the mapping strategy reveals a QTL containing dozens or even hundreds of candidate genes that must then be analyzed using conventional molecular biology techniques. Many QTL have been identified with regard to sleep-wake traits (discussed later), indicating substantial genetic control of sleep physiology, but for the most part, the individual genes underlying these traits have eluded identification. To address these limitations, strategies that involve the inclusion of outbred strains of mice, or animals from an ongoing breeding project called the collaborative cross, which involves several phenotypically and genetically diverse strains,[34] are anticipated to greatly enhance the power of this approach. The wider genetic diversity in these animals is expected to permit more precise genetic mapping, resulting in smaller genetic loci that contain only one or a few candidate genes, which can then be validated rapidly without the substantial commitment of time and resources needed to assess candidate genes in much larger genomic regions.

Although there is tremendous promise concerning the use of these techniques to dramatically advance the field in the future, current approaches have already produced important results, yielding exciting and unexpected evidence for the role of specific components of the genome in regulating sleep-wake traits. It is beyond the scope of this article to review all QTL studies in rodents (see article by Pompeiano and colleagues[21] for more detail), but several prominent examples are discussed in detail to highlight the usefulness of this approach as well as the major conclusions that have resulted from it.

To identify loci implicated in the homeostatic regulation of NREM sleep, a RI approach was undertaken. RI strains of mice are created with 20 generations of matings between F2 siblings derived from 2 inbred parental strains. This essentially achieves full homozygosity for the unique set of recombinations occurring in the original F2 progeny. In this way, several recombinant strains were generated from C57BL/6 and DBA/2 parental strains (BXD RI strains). The BXD RI strains underwent EEG analysis to identify QTLs associated with NREM EEG delta power achieved after 6 hours of sleep deprivation.[31,35] Analysis of NREM delta power responses to sleep deprivation revealed that approximately 37% of the total variance in this trait between the strains was explained by genetic factors. Furthermore, a QTL on chromosome 13 accounted for almost half of this genetic variance, suggesting the presence of an important gene. This locus was named dps-1 (delta-power-sleep-1) and subsequently shown to contain the *Homer1* gene, which (discussed previously) encodes a protein implicated in glutamate neurotransmission and intracellular calcium homeostasis.[30] These results suggest that phenotypic variants of *Homer1a* may explain the effects of the identified QTL, highlighting *Homer1a* as an excellent candidate gene contributing to the homeostatic regulation of sleep.

A separate QTL that contributes to the slow delta oscillations (1–4 Hz) that are a hallmark of NREM sleep was also identified in the same BXD RI strains.[36] The data from this study demonstrated that the majority of the variance could be explained by a single locus. A panel of 30 different inbred strains was then examined using a series of markers in the region of chromosome 14 corresponding to the site of the QTL. A single biallelic marker was identified and each of the different strains was classified as having 1 of the 2 possible alleles (B type and D type). A group of divergent strains all having the D allele were subsequently analyzed for EEG activity and shown to possess the predicted EEG properties (power in the theta band [6–7 Hz] divided by the power in the delta band) associated with that particular allele. Additional polymorphic markers were then used across these strains to narrow this genomic region to approximately 350 kb, which was shown to contain the gene for retinoic acid receptor beta (*Rarb*).[36]

Rarb contains a restriction fragment length polymorphism that completely cosegregates with the genetic marker used to predict the trait. Molecular analysis, including sequencing and targeted deletion studies, was then used to clearly demonstrate that *Rarb* alleles were responsible for the trait. Retinoic acid receptors are widely expressed in the brain and have been implicated in a range of neuronal functions, including long-term potentiation, control of locomotion, and the regulation of dopaminergic and cholinergic neurotransmission.[37] Different *Rarb* alleles may, therefore, have specific effects on aspects of neurotransmission that could potentially lead to altered patterns of neuronal firing that underlie synchronous cortical activity, which is ultimately responsible for the activity within the delta and theta bands.

Similar methodology was used by the same group of researchers to identify acyl-coenzyme A dehydrogenase (*Acads*) as a major gene involved in regulating the frequency of theta oscillations during REM sleep (**Fig. 1**).[38] BALB/cByJ mice, which harbor a mutation in *Acads*,[39] a gene encoding the enzyme that catalyzes the first step in the β-oxidation of C_4-C_6 fatty acids, exhibit a significant reduction in theta frequency, specifically during REM sleep. Furthermore, these mice also have increased expression of *Glo1* (Glyoxylase 1), an enzyme that participates in metabolic byproduct detoxification.[38] These findings implicate metabolic pathways involving fatty acid β-oxidation in regulating theta oscillations during sleep, providing an unexpected, yet profound, molecular link between cellular metabolism and REM sleep regulation.

In a different study recently undertaken, a comprehensive analysis of 20 different sleep-wake traits, grouped into 5 categories (fragmentation, REM sleep, state amount, power bands, and latency), in 269 mice from a segregating population was completed. At least 20 genomic loci, containing 52 significant QTL, were identified as regulators of many diverse sleep-wake traits (**Fig. 2**).[40] Twenty-eight of these QTL were specific for individual traits (eg, duration of REM sleep) over a 24-hour day, whereas others influenced the trait during only the light or dark period or had opposing effects on the trait during the light versus the dark phase. In order to accurately analyze this large data set, a systems biology approach was undertaken and has revealed complex and unexpected results. For example, the seemingly different sleep-wake traits of REM latency and the number of arousals seem regulated, at least in part, by shared genetic mechanisms. Also, there is evidence suggesting that the number and duration of REM bouts, 2 traits previously expected to be highly related, are under differential genetic control.[40]

Although the identity of the individual genes underlying these QTL remains to be determined, these results demonstrate that a complex genetic landscape underlies and regulates many sleep-wake traits. In addition, future studies can integrate gene expression data with these results through an extension of the QTL approach, termed *expression QTL (eQTL) analysis*, which treats variation in the amounts of expressed transcripts as quantifiable traits. By determining which genomic loci are responsible for the regulation of transcription levels of certain genes, eQTL analysis provides a powerful opportunity to examine the relationships between the genome, the transcriptome, and the behavior or phenotype of interest. Furthermore, statistical testing can be used to infer the directionality of these relationships to predict which expressed transcripts causally regulate the phenotype of interest. These results and potential future experimental directions emphasize that a systems

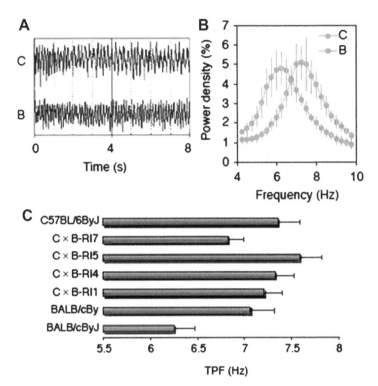

Fig. 1. A mutation in *Acads* is responsible for strain differences in theta peak frequency (TPF) during REM sleep. (*A*) Representative EEG samples during REM sleep in individual BALB/cByJ (C) and C57BL/6J (B) mice. (*B*) Density analysis of EEG spectra ($\pm$1 SD) in the theta range (5–9 Hz) indicates that TPF is 1 Hz faster in B mice (n = 10 per genotype). (*C*) TPF during REM sleep (mean + SD) in parental and recombinant-inbred strains. C, BALB/cBy; B, C57BL/6ByJ. TPF in all C $\times$ B recombinant-inbred strains (and their parental C57BL/6ByJ and BALB/cBy strains) was faster than in BALB/cByJ mice (ANOVA, $F_{6,45}$ = 31.55; $P<2 \times 10^{-12}$; Scheffé test, $P<.01$),[38] which are known to harbor a mutation in *Acads*. Thus, disrupted *Acads* is responsible for the decreased frequency of theta oscillations during REM sleep in these mice. (*Adapted from* Tafti M, Petit B, Chollet D, et al. Deficiency in short-chain fatty acid beta-oxidation affects theta oscillations during sleep. Nat Genet 2003;34:320–5; with permission.)

biology approach may be informative in developing a more complete understanding of how individual genes act as components of networks of interacting molecules that collectively give rise to complex behaviors, such as sleep.

In summary, QTL studies in mice have begun to uncover genomic loci and even individual genes implicated in the regulation of sleep-wake traits. It is important to recognize that in spite of decades of research exploring sleep-wake properties in rodents, much remains to be learned about which genes are involved in regulating sleep and how those molecules specifically affect sleep-wake physiology. The complexity of sleep as well as the dramatic influence of many pharmacologic agents and environmental factors on sleep-wake parameters suggests that many genes and gene networks are involved in controlling sleep. Technologic advances in genetic mapping using different strains of mice, high-throughput sleep recording abilities, and complex computational biology

approaches are expected to further understanding of the genetic basis of sleep, which remains important from a medical as well as a biologic perspective.

KNOCKOUT, TRANSGENIC, AND MUTAGENESIS APPROACHES IN THE MOUSE
Reverse Genetics

Strategies exploring the phenotypic effects of targeted, selective disruption of specific genes are referred to as reverse genetics approaches because the progression is from genotype to phenotype.[41] Basically, this approach uses knockout and transgenic technologies in the mouse to specifically ablate the gene of interest, and the phenotype or behavior under investigation is then measured in animals lacking that particular gene.[42,43] Advances in transgenic technologies and targeted deletion of individual genes in mice have contributed significantly to our understanding of the role of specific genes in sleep

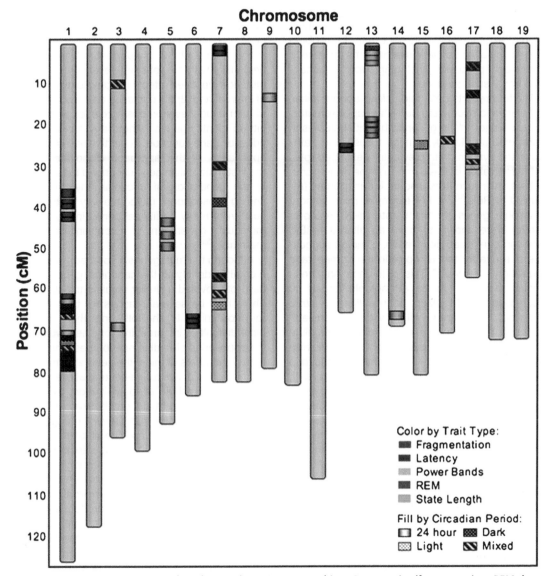

Fig. 2. A comprehensive analysis of 20 sleep-wake traits, grouped into 5 categories (fragmentation, REM sleep, state amount, power bands, and latency), in 269 mice from a segregating population reveals at least 20 genomic loci, containing 52 significant QTL, as responsible for variation in these traits. The colored bands represented the peak logarithm of the odds (LOD) score for each QTL and the fill of the bands indicates the time period for trait linkage, as shown in the insert legend. (*From* Winrow CJ, Williams DL, Kasarskis A, et al. Uncovering the genetic landscape for multiple sleep-wake traits. PLoS One 2009;4:e5161.)

physiology (reviewed in Refs.[35,44]). One important consideration that complicates the interpretation of studies using these techniques is developmental compensation. It may be possible for different genes, perhaps from the same or similar gene families, to perform the function of the missing protein.[45] Thus, some studies may miss the effects of specific genes whose functions may be performed by similar genes still present. Also, there may be additional, nonspecific effects caused by removal of the gene of interest from tissues other than those directly controlling the trait under investigation.

To address these issues, the development and use of animals genetically engineered to eliminate genes at particular times and/or in specific tissues only (termed conditional-knockout or inducible-knockout animals) are important to make accurate conclusions about the precise functions of individual genes in certain tissues and/or structures of interest in relation to the regulation of sleep. Another concern that must be considered in these studies is the effect of genetic background. In spite of these limitations, these techniques remain integral experimental tools necessary for probing the molecular and genetic mechanisms underlying physiologic processes, including complex behavioral traits, such as sleep.

The first reports describing sleep abnormalities in transgenic mice were published approximately 15 years ago.[46,47] In general, the initial studies in transgenic and knockout mice focused on pathways and systems with previously described roles in the regulation of sleep: monoamine neurotransmitters, their receptors, and their transporters (reviewed in Refs.[35,44]). For example, mice without functional genes for the serotonin-2C receptor (Htr2c) were shown to have an altered NREM rebound after sleep deprivation, a finding suggestive of a role for this receptor in the homeostatic regulation of sleep.[48] This difference has been shown, however, to be attributable largely to decreased NREM sleep at baseline in Htr2c knockout compared with wild-type mice.[21] Although this receptor may not directly regulate the response to sleep deprivation or the maintenance of homeostasis, it does seem to influence the endogenous regulation of sleep. Similarly, mice lacking the 1A and 1B subtypes of the serotonin receptor (Htr1a and Htr1b, respectively) exhibit increased levels of REM sleep at baseline (and after 6 hours of sleep deprivation),[49,50] further implicating these receptors and the serotonergic system, in general. Additionally, several studies have conclusively demonstrated a role for cytokines (including interleukin-1, interleukin-10, and tumor necrosis factor) and their receptors in sleep physiology.[51]

Forward Genetics

In contrast to moving from genotype to phenotype, forward genetics entails a progression from phenotype to genotype.[41] For example, the QTL approach for gene identification is considered a forward genetics approach because measurements of the variation in a phenotype of interest are taken first and then used in conjunction with DNA sequence data to determine the underlying genetic loci involved in the regulation of that phenotype. Another forward genetics approach uses mutations induced randomly in the genome using techniques or compounds, such as chemical mutagens, that interfere with DNA in nonspecific ways. The mutagen is applied to a population of animals who are then screened for particular abnormalities related to the phenotype of interest. Then, once mutants are identified, the animals are bred in an attempt to determine the mode of inheritance, map the location of the mutation in the genome, and ultimately clone the underlying gene.

This approach has important advantages: (1) beginning with the phenotype ensures that any mutation identified affects the physiologic process of interest and (2) the unbiased and random nature of the mutagenesis process provides an opportunity to identify genes without any a priori knowledge of gene function. A particularly successful application of this approach discovered Clock, the first mammalian gene described to be involved in the generation of circadian rhythms.[52] This finding subsequently paved the way for the identification of many additional genes involved in the molecular generation of circadian rhythms in mammals.[53]

Although the mutagenesis approach was instrumental in identifying the canonical gene, Clock, it has not provided a similar result in the sleep field. There may be several reasons for this, including (but not limited to) the following: there are technical difficulties in screening for sleep-wake traits (as opposed to circadian phenotypes for example) in large numbers of mice; the generated mutations may produce only subtle effects that are currently below the threshold of identification; the effects may be influenced by genetic background and/or epistatic interactions that prevent recognition of the altered phenotype; and the inherent variability in the phenotype may mask the effects of certain mutations. The mutagenesis approach is probably most appropriate for mutations that are fully penetrant and behave according to mendelian predictions. In contrast, the QTL approach is perhaps best suited to determine which genomic loci underlie natural phenotypic variation within populations of animals and the networks of genes that collectively control sleep-wake traits.

GENETIC DISRUPTION OF CIRCADIAN RHYTHMS INVARIABLY LEADS TO ALTERATIONS IN SLEEP

In conjunction with transgenic and knockout studies (described previously), a large body of evidence from studies exploring sleep-wake traits in mice with mutations in or targeted knockout of canonical circadian clock genes have conclusively demonstrated an integral role of the circadian system in the regulation of sleep (**Table 1**).[54] In addition to affecting temporal patterns of sleep, genetic components of the circadian system influence many other aspects of sleep, including its homeostatic regulation. For example, Clock-mutant mice have significantly reduced amounts of NREM sleep at baseline. In addition, when

Table 1
Sleep-wake patterns in animal models of circadian clock gene disruption

Circadian Mutant/Knock-out	Baseline 24-Hour Wake Percentage	Baseline 24-Hour NREM Percentage	Baseline 24-Hour REM Percentage	Baseline Sleep Fragmentation	Baseline NREM Delta Activity	Recovery Response NREM Activity[a]	Source
Clock	↑	↓	—	—	—	—	55
Npas2	↑	↓	↓	—	—	—	60
Npas2	↑	↓	—	—	—	↓	91
Bmal1	↓	↑	↑	↑	↑	↓	61
Cry1/Cry2	↓	↑	↑	↓	↑	↓	56
Per1	—	—	—	—	—	↓	58
Per1	—	—	—	—	—	↑	59
Per2	—	—	—	—	—	↓	58
Per2	—	—	—	—	—	—	59
Per3	—	—	—	—	—	—	59
Per1/Per2	—	—	—	—	—	↑	59

Circadian clock mutant and deficient mice compared with wild-type mice. Empty cells indicate that information was not presented for the respective trait or could not be clearly interpreted. Many different sleep-deprivation paradigms and data analysis formats were used in these studies, making it difficult to directly compare the recovery sleep patterns among many of the animal models. ↑, increase; ↓, decrease; —, no change.

[a] In the first few hours after sleep deprivation; recovery response in NREM EEG delta power is the standard measurement of sleep homeostatic drive.

Reprinted from Laposky AD, Turek FW. Circadian genes and the sleep-wake cycle. In: Squire LR, editor. Encyclopedia of neuroscience. Oxford (UK): Academic Press; 2009. p. 909–14; with permission.

compared with wild-type animals, they exhibit a smaller compensatory increase in REM sleep after deprivation.[55] *Cry1/Cry2* double knockout mice exhibit signs of increased NREM sleep pressure, such as greater NREM sleep amount, increased NREM sleep consolidation, and elevated NREM sleep delta power, all under baseline conditions.[56] These results indicate that *Clock* and the *Cry* genes have roles in regulating aspects of sleep duration and homeostasis in addition to their function in the generation and maintenance of circadian rhythms.

The expression of the *Per* genes (*Per1, Per2,* and *Per3*) is controlled in part by activity of the *Cry* genes.[53] *Per1* and *Per2* have also been shown to be up-regulated in response to sleep deprivation,[57] suggesting a potential role in sleep homeostasis. Independent experiments examining single *Per1*, *Per2*, and *Per3* knockout mice, as well as double *Per1/Per2* knockout mice, documented a range of sleep-related changes in these animals, but the investigators concluded that there were not any substantial effects on sleep homeostasis.[58,59] Several of the sleep alterations in these animals do not seem, however, to be circadian in nature (eg, *Per1* knockouts and *Per1/Per2* double knockouts have a longer period of elevated delta power after sleep deprivation). Furthermore, *Per* mutations, in addition to affecting the timing of sleep, influence total sleep time as well as the effects of light and dark on sleep.[21] Taken together, these results are consistent with a role for the *Per* genes in specific sleep-related processes in addition to their function in regulating circadian rhythms and the timing of sleep. Finally, it is important to remember that there are 3 mammalian *Per* genes, thus compensation for the specific genes knocked-out may be sufficient to prevent more dramatic changes in sleep-wake regulation from being observed.

Additional evidence for the role of the circadian clock and circadian clock genes in the regulation of sleep homeostasis comes from studies in *Npas2*-deficient and *Bmal*-deficient mice[60,61] as well as from studies of animals with lesions of the central circadian clock, located in the suprachiasmatic nucleus (SCN) in the hypothalamus. Although initial studies in rats suggested that the contribution of the circadian clock in the SCN to the homeostatic regulation of sleep was minimal, if even present,[62,63] subsequent work in SCN-lesioned mice[64] and monkeys[65] has demonstrated that the intact SCN can influence the amount of sleep as well as the temporal control of sleep and wake. Further evidence implicating the circadian system and clock genes in specific sleep-wake processes comes from studies in *Drosophila*.[10]

The profound connection between circadian rhythms and sleep is perhaps best understood from an evolutionary perspective. Circadian rhythms and sleep may have evolved together to coordinate and execute the temporal behavioral, biochemical, molecular, and physiologic program of the organism.[66] Therefore, it should not be surprising that the genetic regulation of circadian rhythms overlaps significantly with that of sleep. The observation that significant sleep abnormalities are present in animals harboring genetic disruptions of the circadian system (see **Table 1**) supports the hypothesis that sleep and circadian rhythms are under shared genetic control. It is important to point out that this article is not arguing that all genes involved in controlling sleep-wake traits are circadian nor that all genetic components of the circadian system directly influence the sleep-wake cycle. These significant genetic relationships between circadian rhythms and sleep-wake physiology are simply framed within their potential evolutionary basis.

THE GENETICS OF SLEEP OFFER A UNIQUE LINK TO THE GENETICS OF CHRONIC DISEASE

The observation that circadian rhythms and sleep are highly intertwined at the genetic and molecular levels has special importance in the context of recent findings linking circadian rhythms to a range of chronic metabolic[15] and cardiovascular[14] diseases of critical importance to public health. Circadian mutant and knockout animals have emerged as important models for diseases, such as the metabolic syndrome,[67] diabetes,[68] and hypertension,[69] among others, implying that the common genetic mechanisms underlying sleep and circadian rhythms are intimately related to these pervasive chronic diseases. In addition, growing experimental and epidemiologic evidence indicates that reduced and/or poor quality sleep is an independent risk factor for metabolic and cardiovascular disease (reviewed by Spiegel and coworkers[16]). In spite of these observations, there are few mechanistic hypotheses to explain exactly how disturbed circadian rhythms and/or sleep contributes to or influences the development of these diseases, which are traditionally considered peripheral in nature.

Although dysfunction in peripheral organs (adipose tissue, pancreas, liver, and so forth) is undoubtedly important to the pathogenesis of these diseases, it is reasonable to hypothesize that the CNS also serves a crucial role. Circadian rhythm and/or sleep disruption may negatively affect the CNS' ability to regulate metabolic processes necessary to maintain homeostasis and prevent disease development under certain environmental conditions. An intriguing possibility is that one function of sleep may be to monitor and regulate energy balance at the molecular level within the brain.[70] Components of the circadian system have also recently been shown to be sensitive to redox state within the cell, potentially linking circadian rhythms and basic energy metabolism.[71,72] Therefore, disruptions of sleep and/or circadian rhythms may hinder the ability of the CNS to accurately regulate metabolic processes and energy balance within in the CNS and possibly throughout the organism, which may predispose individuals to the development of metabolic and/or cardiovascular disease. Although many details concerning the generation and regulation of circadian rhythms are understood at the molecular level,[53] there are many outstanding questions regarding understanding of the physiologic and molecular processes underlying sleep that remain to be answered. Studies that continue to elucidate the genetic basis of its regulation are expected to contribute to understanding of how sleep is working at the molecular level, which, when integrated with understanding of circadian rhythms, may provide insight into the pathogenesis and progression of certain metabolic and cardiovascular diseases shown to be linked to disturbed circadian rhythms and/or sleep.

Similarly, both circadian rhythm and sleep disturbances have been extensively implicated in psychiatric and neurodegenerative disease.[13] For example, the *Clock* mutant mouse was originally shown to exhibit anxiety-like behavior,[73] and, on further investigation, has emerged as a potential model for mania-like behavior.[74] An understanding of the circadian system seems relevant for bipolar disorders in humans.[75] Also, recent evidence suggests that normalization of sleep-wake cycles and circadian patterns of activity may be beneficial in a transgenic mouse model of Huntington disease.[76] These are only a few of the many examples of how the regulation of circadian rhythms, which are tightly coupled to the generation of normal sleep-wake cycles,[66] at both the genetic and environmental levels is implicated in psychiatric and neurodegenerative disease pathology and pathogenesis.

Perhaps the strongest evidence linking neuropsychiatric disease to sleep specifically occurs in depression.[77] The overwhelming majority of patients with depression experience sleep-wake disturbances (as many as 90% in some studies[78]). Furthermore, periods of insomnia often precede episodes of depression,[79] and successful treatment of insomnia often decreases the length, severity, and incidence of clinical depressive episodes.[80] Depressed patients also experience circadian rhythm disturbances,[81,82] which likely occur in unison with the sleep-wake abnormalities. The intimate neuroanatomic, physiologic, and genetic connections between sleep and circadian rhythms[66] support the hypothesis that dysfunction of sleep-wake cycles leads to reciprocal disturbances in the circadian system, which then leads to increased sleep-wake abnormalities, creating a vicious cycle. There are several hypotheses about the mechanistic basis of the relationship between sleep, circadian rhythms, and depression that are beyond the scope of this article (reviewed in Refs.[83–85]), but strong experimental support is lacking. Studies in animal models are essential to refine and provide collaborative evidence and support for these hypotheses, and examination of the genetic basis of sleep-wake traits should provide unique insight into individual molecules, pathways, and genetic networks that may be implicated in the pathogenesis of depression as well as other psychiatric and neurodegenerative disorders.

The animal models and clinical evidence described above represent a few examples of specific disease processes associated with sleep and circadian rhythms. Due to the highly conserved evolutionary basis of the crucial processes of sleep and circadian rhythms, they are expected to be involved in nearly all aspects of central and peripheral physiology and, therefore, implicated in the pathogenesis of many other diseases as well. As a testament to just how highly intertwined sleep and circadian rhythms are, with few exceptions, most studies have failed to separate the effects of circadian rhythm disturbances, specifically from those caused by sleep loss. For example, although it has traditionally been assumed that the increased incidence of chronic diseases in shift workers is due to circadian disruption,[86–88] it has never been shown that it is not due to sleep disturbances, which are also exceedingly common in these individuals.[89] Therefore, the fundamental connection between circadian rhythms and sleep should not be overlooked, and more work needs to be done to separate the effects of circadian disturbances versus sleep restriction as well as any synergistic effects that may arise.

SUMMARY

In summary, animal models have played a significant role in understanding of the genetic basis of sleep. In addition to verifying the roles of key neurotransmitter systems in sleep physiology, animal models have revealed important functions for previously unsuspected genes, such as those involved in fatty acid metabolism and β-oxidation. For decades, it has been known that many aspects of sleep are under substantial genetic control, and several studies have reported many specific genomic loci that are associated with individual traits. Much work remains, however, to conclusively identify the particular genes within those loci as well as the networks of interacting genes that together are responsible for the regulation of specific traits. Future work is expected to identify these individual genes and networks, which will lead to testable hypotheses that can be used by researchers to examine the effects of perturbations of these molecules and networks on sleep-wake regulation and physiology. This will allow scientists to probe the molecular mechanisms underlying sleep and perhaps begin to provide some satisfying answers to the ultimate question of why we sleep. The recent reporting of successful targeted gene knockout strategies using embryonic stem cells in the rat[90] offers an exciting opportunity to study genetics in an animal model more amenable to neuroanatomic manipulation and physiologic experimentation than the mouse. Studies using animal models remain integral to the sleep field and will contribute to advances in understanding of the genetic basis of sleep that may yield unexpected insight into the pathogenesis and development of diseases that have been associated with sleep abnormalities.

REFERENCES

1. Ambrosius U, Lietzenmaier S, Wehrle R, et al. Heritability of sleep electroencephalogram. Biol Psychiatry 2008;64:344–8.
2. De Gennaro L, Marzano C, Fratello F, et al. The electroencephalographic fingerprint of sleep is genetically determined: a twin study. Ann Neurol 2008; 64:455–60.
3. Thompson PM, Cannon TD, Narr KL, et al. Genetic influences on brain structure. Nat Neurosci 2001;4: 1253–8.
4. Stassen HH, Lykken DT, Propping P, et al. Genetic determination of the human EEG. Survey of recent results on twins reared together and apart. Hum Genet 1988;80:165–76.
5. Tafti M, Maret S, Dauvilliers Y. Genes for normal sleep and sleep disorders. Ann Med 2005;37:580–9.
6. Kitahama K, Valatx JL. Instrumental and pharmacological paradoxical sleep deprivation in mice: strain differences. Neuropharmacology 1980;19:529–35.
7. Valatx JL. Possible embryonic origin of sleep interstrain differences in the mouse. Prog Brain Res 1978;48:385–91.
8. Valatx JL, Bugat R, Jouvet M. Genetic studies of sleep in mice. Nature 1972;238:226–7.
9. Lin L, Faraco J, Li R, et al. The sleep disorder canine narcolepsy is caused by a mutation in the hypocretin (orexin) receptor 2 gene. Cell 1999;98:365–76.
10. Allada R. Genetics of sleep in a simple model organism: Drosophila. In: Krieger MH, Roth T, Dement WC, editors. Principles and practice of sleep medicine. 5th edition. St Louis (MO): Elsevier Saunders; 2010. p. 151–60.
11. Andretic R, Franken P, Tafti M. Genetics of sleep. Annu Rev Genet 2008;42:361–88.
12. Shaw PJ, Franken P. Perchance to dream: solving the mystery of sleep through genetic analysis. J Neurobiol 2003;54:179–202.
13. Wulff K, Gatti S, Wettstein JG, et al. Sleep and circadian rhythm disruption in psychiatric and neurodegenerative disease. Nat Rev Neurosci 2010;11: 589–99.
14. Durgan DJ, Young ME. The cardiomyocyte circadian clock: emerging roles in health and disease. Circ Res 2010;106:647–58.
15. Green CB, Takahashi JS, Bass J. The meter of metabolism. Cell 2008;134:728–42.
16. Spiegel K, Tasali E, Leproult R, et al. Effects of poor and short sleep on glucose metabolism and obesity risk. Nat Rev Endocrinol 2009;5:253–61.
17. Grassi-Zucconi G, Giuditta A, Mandile P, et al. c-fos spontaneous expression during wakefulness is reversed during sleep in neuronal subsets of the rat cortex. J Physiol Paris 1994;88:91–3.
18. O'Hara BF, Young KA, Watson FL, et al. Immediate early gene expression in brain during sleep deprivation: preliminary observations. Sleep 1993;16:1–7.
19. Pompeiano M, Cirelli C, Tononi G. Immediate-early genes in spontaneous wakefulness and sleep: expression of c-fos and NGFI-A mRNA and protein. J Sleep Res 1994;3:80–96.
20. Gerashchenko D, Wisor JP, Burns D, et al. Identification of a population of sleep-active cerebral cortex neurons. Proc Natl Acad Sci U S A 2008;105: 10227–32.
21. O'Hara BF, Turek FW, Franken P. Genetic basis of sleep in rodents. In: Principles and practice of sleep medicine. 5th edition. St Louis (MO): Elsevier Saunders; 2010. p. 161–74.
22. Sherin JE, Shiromani PJ, McCarley RW, et al. Activation of ventrolateral preoptic neurons during sleep. Science 1996;271:216–9.
23. Sherin JE, Elmquist JK, Torrealba F, et al. Innervation of histaminergic tuberomammillary neurons by GABAergic and galaninergic neurons in the ventrolateral preoptic nucleus of the rat. J Neurosci 1998;18:4705–21.
24. Saper CB, Scammell TE, Lu J. Hypothalamic regulation of sleep and circadian rhythms. Nature 2005; 437:1257–63.

25. Nakanishi H, Sun Y, Nakamura RK, et al. Positive correlations between cerebral protein synthesis rates and deep sleep in Macaca mulatta. Eur J Neurosci 1997;9:271–9.

26. Ramm P, Smith CT. Rates of cerebral protein synthesis are linked to slow wave sleep in the rat. Physiol Behav 1990;48:749–53.

27. Cirelli C, Gutierrez CM, Tononi G. Extensive and divergent effects of sleep and wakefulness on brain gene expression. Neuron 2004;41:35–43.

28. Mackiewicz M, Shockley KR, Romer MA, et al. Macromolecule biosynthesis: a key function of sleep. Physiol Genomics 2007;31:441–57.

29. Maret S, Dorsaz S, Gurcel L, et al. Homer1a is a core brain molecular correlate of sleep loss. Proc Natl Acad Sci U S A 2007;104:20090–5.

30. Xiao B, Tu JC, Worley PF. Homer: a link between neural activity and glutamate receptor function. Curr Opin Neurobiol 2000;10:370–4.

31. Franken P, Chollet D, Tafti M. The homeostatic regulation of sleep need is under genetic control. J Neurosci 2001;21:2610–21.

32. Wang Z, Gerstein M, Snyder M. RNA-Seq: a revolutionary tool for transcriptomics. Nat Rev Genet 2009; 10:57–63.

33. Flint J, Valdar W, Shifman S, et al. Strategies for mapping and cloning quantitative trait genes in rodents. Nat Rev Genet 2005;6:271–86.

34. Churchill GA, Airey DC, Allayee H, et al. The collaborative cross, a community resource for the genetic analysis of complex traits. Nat Genet 2004;36: 1133–7.

35. Franken P, Tafti M. Genetics of sleep and sleep disorders. Front Biosci 2003;8:e381–97.

36. Maret S, Franken P, Dauvilliers Y, et al. Retinoic acid signaling affects cortical synchrony during sleep. Science 2005;310:111–3.

37. Drager UC. Retinoic acid signaling in the functioning brain. Sci STKE 2006;2006:pe10.

38. Tafti M, Petit B, Chollet D, et al. Deficiency in short-chain fatty acid beta-oxidation affects theta oscillations during sleep. Nat Genet 2003;34:320–5.

39. Reue K, Cohen RD. Acads gene deletion in BALB/cByJ mouse strain occurred after 1981 and is not present in BALB/cByJ-fld mutant mice. Mamm Genome 1996;7:694–5.

40. Winrow CJ, Williams DL, Kasarskis A, et al. Uncovering the genetic landscape for multiple sleep-wake traits. PLoS One 2009;4:e5161.

41. Takahashi JS, Pinto LH, Vitaterna MH. Forward and reverse genetic approaches to behavior in the mouse. Science 1994;264:1724–33.

42. Capecchi MR. The new mouse genetics: altering the genome by gene targeting. Trends Genet 1989;5: 70–6.

43. Jaenisch R. Transgenic animals. Science 1988;240: 1468–74.

44. Wisor JP, Kilduff TS. Molecular genetic advances in sleep research and their relevance to sleep medicine. Sleep 2005;28:357–67.

45. Moran TH, Reeves RH, Rogers D, et al. Ain't misbehavin'—it's genetic! Nat Genet 1996;12:115–6.

46. Tobler I, Gaus SE, Deboer T, et al. Altered circadian activity rhythms and sleep in mice devoid of prion protein. Nature 1996;380:639–42.

47. Zhang J, Obal F Jr, Fang J, et al. Non-rapid eye movement sleep is suppressed in transgenic mice with a deficiency in the somatotropic system. Neurosci Lett 1996;220:97–100.

48. Frank MG, Stryker MP, Tecott LH. Sleep and sleep homeostasis in mice lacking the 5-HT2c receptor. Neuropsychopharmacology 2002;27:869–73.

49. Boutrel B, Franc B, Hen R, et al. Key role of 5-HT1B receptors in the regulation of paradoxical sleep as evidenced in 5-HT1B knock-out mice. J Neurosci 1999;19:3204–12.

50. Boutrel B, Monaca C, Hen R, et al. Involvement of 5-HT1A receptors in homeostatic and stress-induced adaptive regulations of paradoxical sleep: studies in 5-HT1A knock-out mice. J Neurosci 2002;22: 4686–92.

51. Krueger JM, Obal FJ, Fang J, et al. The role of cytokines in physiological sleep regulation. Ann N Y Acad Sci 2001;933:211–21.

52. Vitaterna MH, King DP, Chang AM, et al. Mutagenesis and mapping of a mouse gene, Clock, essential for circadian behavior. Science 1994;264: 719–25.

53. Lowrey PL, Takahashi JS. Mammalian circadian biology: elucidating genome-wide levels of temporal organization. Annu Rev Genomics Hum Genet 2004; 5:407–41.

54. Laposky AD, Turek FW. Circadian genes and the sleep-wake cycle. In: Squire LR, editor. Encyclopedia of neuroscience. Oxford (United Kingdom): Academic Press; 2009. p. 909–14.

55. Naylor E, Bergmann BM, Krauski K, et al. The circadian clock mutation alters sleep homeostasis in the mouse. J Neurosci 2000;20:8138–43.

56. Wisor JP, O'Hara BF, Terao A, et al. A role for cryptochromes in sleep regulation. BMC Neurosci 2002; 3:20.

57. Wisor JP, Pasumarthi RK, Gerashchenko D, et al. Sleep deprivation effects on circadian clock gene expression in the cerebral cortex parallel electroencephalographic differences among mouse strains. J Neurosci 2008;28:7193–201.

58. Kopp C, Albrecht U, Zheng B, et al. Homeostatic sleep regulation is preserved in mPer1 and mPer2 mutant mice. Eur J Neurosci 2002;16:1099–106.

59. Shiromani PJ, Xu M, Winston EM, et al. Sleep rhythmicity and homeostasis in mice with targeted disruption of mPeriod genes. Am J Physiol Regul Integr Comp Physiol 2004;287:R47–57.

60. Dudley CA, Erbel-Sieler C, Estill SJ, et al. Altered patterns of sleep and behavioral adaptability in NPAS2-deficient mice. Science 2003;301:379–83.

61. Laposky A, Easton A, Dugovic C, et al. Deletion of the mammalian circadian clock gene BMAL1/Mop3 alters baseline sleep architecture and the response to sleep deprivation. Sleep 2005;28:395–409.

62. Mistlberger RE, Bergmann BM, Waldenar W, et al. Recovery sleep following sleep deprivation in intact and suprachiasmatic nuclei-lesioned rats. Sleep 1983;6:217–33.

63. Tobler I, Borbely AA, Groos G. The effect of sleep deprivation on sleep in rats with suprachiasmatic lesions. Neurosci Lett 1983;42:49–54.

64. Easton A, Meerlo P, Bergmann B, et al. The suprachiasmatic nucleus regulates sleep timing and amount in mice. Sleep 2004;27:1307–18.

65. Edgar DM, Dement WC, Fuller CA. Effect of SCN lesions on sleep in squirrel monkeys: evidence for opponent processes in sleep-wake regulation. J Neurosci 1993;13:1065–79.

66. Turek FW, Dugovic C, Laposky AD. Master circadian clock, master circadian rhythm. In: Kryger MH, Roth T, Dement WC, editors. Principles and practice of sleep medicine. 4th edition. Philadelphia: Elsevier Saunders; 2005. p. 318–20.

67. Turek FW, Joshu C, Kohsaka A, et al. Obesity and metabolic syndrome in circadian Clock mutant mice. Science 2005;308:1043–5.

68. Marcheva B, Ramsey KM, Buhr ED, et al. Disruption of the clock components CLOCK and BMAL1 leads to hypoinsulinaemia and diabetes. Nature 2010;466:627–31.

69. Doi M, Takahashi Y, Komatsu R, et al. Salt-sensitive hypertension in circadian clock-deficient Cry-null mice involves dysregulated adrenal Hsd3b6. Nat Med 2010;16:67–74.

70. Scharf MT, Naidoo N, Zimmerman JE, et al. The energy hypothesis of sleep revisited. Prog Neurobiol 2008;86:264–80.

71. Reick M, Garcia JA, Dudley C, et al. NPAS2: an analog of clock operative in the mammalian forebrain. Science 2001;293:506–9.

72. Rutter J, Reick M, Wu LC, et al. Regulation of clock and NPAS2 DNA binding by the redox state of NAD cofactors. Science 2001;293:510–4.

73. Easton A, Arbuzova J, Turek FW. The circadian Clock mutation increases exploratory activity and escape-seeking behavior. Genes Brain Behav 2003;2:11–9.

74. Roybal K, Theobold D, Graham A, et al. Mania-like behavior induced by disruption of CLOCK. Proc Natl Acad Sci U S A 2007;104:6406–11.

75. McClung CA. Role for the Clock gene in bipolar disorder. Cold Spring Harb Symp Quant Biol 2007;72:637–44.

76. Pallier PN, Morton AJ. Management of sleep/wake cycles improves cognitive function in a transgenic mouse model of Huntington's disease. Brain Res 2009;1279:90–8.

77. Benca RM. Mood disorders. In: Kryger MH, Roth T, Dement WC, editors. Principles and practice of sleep medicine. Philadelphia: Saunders; 2005. p. 1311–26.

78. Thase ME. Antidepressant treatment of the depressed patient with insomnia. J Clin Psychiatry 1999;60(Suppl 17):28–31 [discussion: 46–8].

79. Perlis ML, Giles DE, Buysse DJ, et al. Self-reported sleep disturbance as a prodromal symptom in recurrent depression. J Affect Disord 1997;42:209–12.

80. Kupfer DJ. Pathophysiology and management of insomnia during depression. Ann Clin Psychiatry 1999;11:267–76.

81. Germain A, Kupfer DJ. Circadian rhythm disturbances in depression. Hum Psychopharmacol 2008;23:571–85.

82. Turek FW. From circadian rhythms to clock genes in depression. Int Clin Psychopharmacol 2007;22(Suppl 2):S1–8.

83. Srinivasan V, Pandi-Perumal SR, Trakht I, et al. Pathophysiology of depression: role of sleep and the melatonergic system. Psychiatry Res 2009;165:201–14.

84. Summa KC, Turek FW. Circadian rhythm disturbances in major depressive disorder. In: Time to enter a new era in depression management. Paris (France): Elsevier Masson; 2010. p. 41–60.

85. Thase ME. Depression and sleep: pathophysiology and treatment. Dialogues Clin Neurosci 2006;8:217–26.

86. Antunes LC, Levandovski R, Dantas G, et al. Obesity and shift work: chronobiological aspects. Nutr Res Rev 2010;23:155–68.

87. Boggild H, Knutsson A. Shift work, risk factors and cardiovascular disease. Scand J Work Environ Health 1999;25:85–99.

88. Knutsson A, Boggild H. Gastrointestinal disorders among shift workers. Scand J Work Environ Health 2010;36:85–95.

89. Akerstedt T. Shift work and disturbed sleep/wakefulness. Occup Med (Lond) 2003;53:89–94.

90. Hamra FK. Gene targeting: enter the rat. Nature 2010;467:161–3.

91. Franken P, Dudley CA, Estill SJ, et al. NPAS2 as a transcriptional regulator of non-rapid eye movement sleep: genotype and sex interactions. Proc Natl Acad Sci U S A 2006;103:7118–23.

Genetics of Electroencephalography During Wakefulness and Sleep

Nathaniel F. Watson, MD, MSc

KEYWORDS

- Genetics • Electroencephalography • Sleep • Twins
- Polymorphism

In 1929, Hans Berger, at the University of Jena in Germany, performed the first recording of electrical activity of the brain and coined the term elektenkephalogram.[1] Through the years, understanding of the electroencephalogram (EEG) has expanded, including characterization of typical frequencies, elucidation of sleep and sleep stages, and appreciation for interictal and ictal phenomena. Today the EEG plays a central role in the diagnosis and treatment of epilepsy and characterization of sleep and sleep disorders.

As an endophenotype of brain activity, the EEG has drawn a substantial amount of interest from researchers attempting to gain a deeper understanding of brain function. Researchers have endeavored to understand the genetic basis of the EEG, in hopes of better conceptualizing the neurophysiologic basis of brain activity. This work originally involved heritability studies in twins, but, with the recent growth in genetic research technologies, it now enters the realm of genomic evaluation. This article summarizes the current state of the genetic aspects of the EEG. Although evoked potentials involve similar neurophysiology as EEG, including these data was beyond the scope of this article.

NEUROPHYSIOLOGY OF ELECTROENCEPHALOGRAPHY

A general understanding of EEG neurophysiology is necessary to fully comprehend the meaning of genetic influences on this phenotype. At its most basic, the EEG measures the electrical potential of a group of neurons located under the scalp, adjacent to the surface electrode placed on the scalp over this region. The nature of the action potential offers a host of cellular mechanisms to consider as the possible method by which genetic variation influences the EEG.

Neurons are electrically polarized by membrane-bound ion channels, resulting in a membrane potential. The membrane potential has 2 important components: the resting potential, representing the potential of the membrane in the undisturbed state (usually close to -70 mV), and the threshold potential, representing the potential more than which there is vigorous conduction of an action potential (usually -55 mV). Neuronal synaptic inputs that depolarize the cell to the threshold potential generate an action potential. This process is extremely short lived and mobile, mediated by voltage-gated ion channels and taking place in less than 0.001 of a second. Membrane potential increase causes opening of sodium ion channels, resulting in intracellular sodium ion influx. The resulting increase in intracellular cations serves to depolarize the cell. Concurrent with this process, opening of potassium ion channels causes potassium efflux from the cell, opposing the sodium-mediated depolarization and hyperpolarizing the cell. During this process, if the membrane potential depolarizes to the threshold potential, then the

Funding: This work was supported by NIH grants K23HL083350-01A1, 5P30NR011400-02, and a University of Washington General Clinical Research Center Pilot Grant.
Conflicts of interest: The author has nothing to disclose.
Department of Neurology and University of Washington Medicine Sleep Center, 325 Ninth Avenue, Box 359803, Seattle, WA 98104-2499, USA
E-mail address: nwatson@uw.edu

Sleep Med Clin 6 (2011) 155–169
doi:10.1016/j.jsmc.2011.04.003

activity of the sodium ion channels dominates and an action potential is generated. On completion of the action potential, efflux of potassium from the cell, along with the activity of the sodium-potassium pump, resets the resting membrane potential. This action potential is the basis of the EEG.[2]

A single action potential cannot generate a scalp EEG reading, just as a pebble dropped in the ocean cannot generate a major wave. Neuronally generated action potentials travel down axons, ultimately resulting in the release of neurotransmitters into the synaptic cleft between 2 neurons. These neurotransmitters stimulate postsynaptic receptors on the dendrite or body of the neighboring cell, generating a postsynaptic current. These currents then summate to generate an action potential. On a microscale, the EEG represents the electrical current within a single dendritic spine. On the macroscale, the EEG reflects the correlated synaptic activity caused by postsynaptic potentials of a massive number of neurons. Furthermore, the postsynaptic potentials captured by surface EEG represent those generated from the superficial layers of the cortex, abutting the skull, because of

dampening of the signal by the meninges, cerebrospinal fluid, and skull. As a result, genetic studies of surface EEG assess a neurophysiologically complex, but neuroanatomically limited, phenotype.

EEG MEASUREMENT AND CATEGORIZATION

EEG signals are acquired via tin, silver, or gold electrodes placed on the scalp with a conductive gel or paste in a traditional 10 to 20 system (**Fig. 1**). Polysomnography (PSG) typically does not include the full array of electrodes, but focuses on 3 derivations for the purposes of staging sleep that include F4-M1, C4-M1, and O2-M1. In general, the digital signal is amplified, passed through an antialiasing filter, and converted from analog to digital with sampling typically occurring at 256 to 512 Hz. There are 2 montages that are most often used: the bipolar, in which each channel represents the difference in voltage between 2 adjacent electrodes, and the referential, in which each channel represents the difference in voltage between a certain electrode and a designated reference electrode. The referential montage is typically used in overnight sleep studies, whereas both the referential

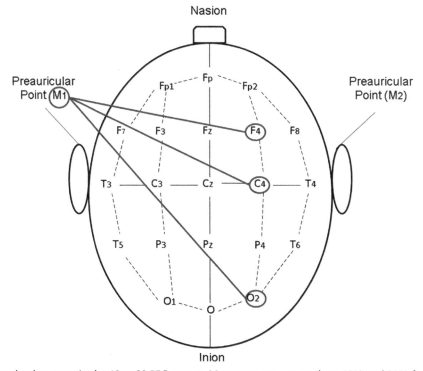

Fig. 1. Electrode placement in the 10 to 20 EEG system. Measurements are made at 10% and 20% from nasion to inion, between the preauricular points, and around the circumference of the head. Measurements from the nasion, inion, and bilateral preauricular points to the closest electrode are 10%, as are measurements from Fp to Fp1 and Fp2 and O to O1 and O2. All other measurements are 20%. The recommended derivations for polysomnography recording are F4-M1, C4-M1, and O2-M1, as indicated in red.

and bipolar montages are used in EEG recordings in the epilepsy setting.

EEG rhythmical activity is divided into bands by frequency. Most scalp EEG signal emanating from the cerebrum is in the range of 1 to 20 Hz, with frequencies greater than and less than this range likely to be artifact. EEG frequency bands are divided into 5 categories based on anatomic distribution and biologic significance. These categories include Δ (up to 4 Hz), θ (4–7 Hz), α (8–12 Hz), σ (12–16 Hz), β (16–30 Hz), and γ (30–100 Hz). Δ Sleep is also known as slow wave sleep (SWS). For sleep staging purposes, the EEG is divided up into non–rapid eye movement (NREM) and rapid eye movement (REM) sleep. NREM sleep is further divided into stages N1 (low-voltage, mixed frequency EEG with slow rolling eye movements), N2 (14-Hz sleep spindles and K-complexes), and N3 (waves 0.5–2 Hz with a peak-to-peak amplitude of at least 75 μV) (**Fig. 2**). Sleep staging and EEG interpretation are both typically scored and interpreted by trained professionals. Power spectral analysis (PSA) is the quantification of EEG power by frequency using a fast Fourier transform. The data are typically broken down into discreet periods of time, and power values are presented in μV^2 (**Fig. 3**). Depth of sleep is often characterized by the Δ power, which refers to the frequency and amplitude of the Δ waves produced as ascertained by PSA. Δ Power is considered representative of the homeostatic drive to sleep, with the higher the power the greater the animal's drive to sleep.[3,4]

THE EEG IN TWIN AND FAMILY STUDIES

The genetic influence on phenotypes such as the EEG can be studied with twin or family studies, in which the resemblance for a trait among family members is compared. monozygotic (MZ) twin pairs are genetically identical to each other, whereas dizygotic (DZ) twins and nontwin siblings

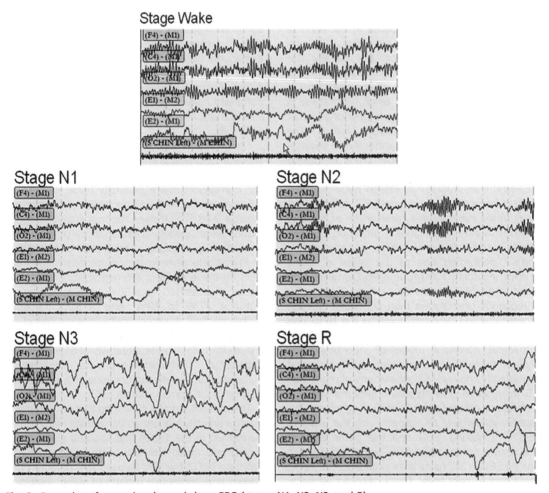

Fig. 2. Examples of normal wake and sleep EEG (stages N1, N2, N3, and R).

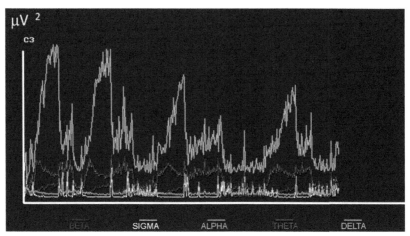

Fig. 3. Example of all-night PSA, Δ (0.5–3.9 Hz), θ (4.0–7.9 Hz), α (8.0–11.9 Hz), σ (12.0–15.9 Hz), and β (16.0–31.9 Hz) bands (x-axis is time). (*Courtesy of* Roseanne Armitage, PhD, Ann Arbor, MI.)

share, on average, 50% of their segregating genes. Environmental factors are believed to be comparable between MZ and DZ twins. Twin studies assessing EEG phenotypes generally use a classic twin study methodology in which the condition of interest is compared in MZ and DZ twin pairs (ie, the intrapair similarity). Although disease-specific mechanisms are usually unknown, heritability can be estimated by examining the difference in disease or phenotype concordance between MZ and DZ twins. Heritability is the proportion of variance in a phenotypic trait that can be attributed to genetic factors.[5] The remainder of the influence is attributed to environmental factors shared by both twins or unique experiences affecting only 1 member of a pair.

Several twin studies have been performed assessing heritability of various EEG parameters. Many of the initial studies focused on aspects of α waves during wakefulness, including α wave activity, index, frequency, and persistence.[6–12] Vogel[13] performed one of the larger of these studies, including 100 MZ and 98 DZ twins, and found that MZ concordance was higher for α frequency phenotypes than DZ twins. He also showed that EEG variants, such as the 16 to 19/s β waves or the low-voltage EEG, follow a mendelian autosomal dominant mode of inheritance.[14,15] Multiple follow-up studies were performed that consistently showed MZ correlations of more than 0.5 for α wave phenotypes, compared with DZ correlations of less than 0.3, confirming substantial genetic influences on aspects of the wakeful EEG.[16,17] Waking EEG spectral patterns have also shown substantial within-pair similarity. The waking EEG in MZ twins is as similar as that of the same person over time. The within-pair similarity of DZ twins is significantly higher than that in

unrelated individuals, and the EEGs of MZ twins reared apart is as similar to each other as are the EEGs of the same person over time or as the EEGs of MZ twins reared together.[18] More recently, α power heritability has been found to be as high as 85%, with variance in frontal asymmetry as high as 28%.[19] Linkage studies in 17 families with 191 individuals determined that a single locus on the human chromosome 20q was associated with a low-voltage EEG variant characterized by near complete absence of α waves.[20] Other than this, little genetic linkage analysis has been done on EEG traits.

Next, researchers expanded their focus of the wakeful EEG spectra from α frequency waves to Δ, θ, and β waves. Again, for all of these spectra, MZ correlations were generally twice as high as DZ correlations, with MZ correlations reaching as high as 0.86.[21–25] Power spectral analytical techniques were applied to obtain more precise EEG phenotyping, resulting in expanded opportunities to investigate genetic factors contributing to the EEG. In these studies, the heritability of absolute power of Δ ranged from 30% to 76%, θ 51% to 89%, α 47% to 89%, and β 52% to 86% (**Table 1**).[26–33] A recent meta-analysis found an average heritability of α power of 79%, with an α peak frequency metaheritability of 81%.[34] These substantial heritabilities provide convincing evidence that genetic factors underlie a substantial portion of the human waking EEG.

The earliest studies indicating that human sleep was genetically influenced came from twin studies performed in the 1930s that showed sleep onset timing and sleep amounts were more similar in MZ than in DZ twins.[35] Subsequent research has shown that subjective reports of sleep, including daytime napping, habitual bedtime, wake time,

Table 1
Twin studies of PSA in the wake EEG

Study	Subjects (Years of Age)	EEG Parameters	Genetic Analysis	Results (h²)
van Beijsterveldt et al,[29] 1996	91 MZ, 122 DZ; (16)	PSA; Δ, θ, α, β	SEM	Δ = 76%; θ = 89%; α = 89%; β = 86%
van Baal et al,[28] 1996	71 MZ, 96 DZ; (5)	PSA; θ, α1, α2, β1, β2	SEM	θ = 81%; α1 = 81%; α2 = 78%; β1 = 73%; β2 = 64%
Christian et al,[27] 1996	53 MZ, 38 DZ; (30)	PSA; θ, α, β	SEM	θ = 62%; α = 59%; β = 40%
van Baal et al,[31] 1998	70 MZ, 97 DZ; (5)	PSA; EEG coherence; θ	SEM	θ = 30%–71%
van Beijsterveldt et al,[30] 1998	91 MZ, 126 DZ; (16)	PSA; EEG coherence; Δ, θ, α, β	SEM	Δ = 30%–56%; θ = 51%–73%; α = 47%–81%; β = 52%–70%
McGuire et al,[26] 1998	33 MZ, 17 DZ (15); 45 MZ, 24 DZ (17)	PSA; θ, α	SEM	(age 15 y); θ = 58–78%; α = 62–78% (age 17 y); θ = 76%–86%; α = 76%–83%
van Baal et al,[32] 2001	70 MZ, 97 DZ; (5 and 7)	PSA; EEG coherence; θ	Longitudinal genetic model	(age 5 y); θ = 53%–75%; (age 7 y); θ = 36%–77%
Posthuma et al,[33] 2001	47 MZ; 253 DZ/sibs; 44 MZ, 192 DZ/sibs	PSA; α peak frequency	SEM with regression of age and gender on mean	Adults 71%, older adults 83%
Gao et al,[19] 2009	951 twins, 9–10	PSA; Frontal EEG asymmetry, α power	SEM	Frontal asymmetry 11%–28%, α power 71%–85%

EEG coherence measures the covariation in electrical brain activity between 2 locations on the scalp.

Abbreviations: DZ, dizygotic; h², heritability; MZ, monozygotic; PSA, power spectral analysis; SEM, structural equation modeling; sibs, siblings.

Adapted from van Beijsterveldt, van Baal GC. Twin and family studies of the human electroencephalogram: a review and meta-analysis. Biol Psychol 2002;61:114–7; with permission from Elsevier.

sleep duration, arousals, and subjective sleep quality, exhibit strong heritability.[36,37] The first twin study to focus on the EEG during sleep was performed in 1966 by Zung and Wilson.[38] They visually inspected the sleep EEG in 4 MZ and 2 DZ pairs and determined substantial concordance between the temporal patterns of sleep stages in MZ compared with DZ twins. Subsequent studies involving sleep recordings in 15 MZ and 9 DZ neonatal twins (40 weeks after conception) found a higher concordance for REM sleep in the MZ twins.[39] In the 1980s, Webb and Campbell[40] recorded sleep in 14 MZ and 14 DZ twin pairs and found that sleep latency, awakening measures, stage changes, and REM amounts were more highly correlated in MZ than in DZ twins. Not long thereafter, REM period length and sleep spindle density were found to be highly correlated in MZ twins.[41,42] This work was expanded in the early 1990s by Linkowski and colleagues,[43,44] who performed 3 consecutive nights of overnight sleep EEG recordings in 11 MZ and 15 DZ twin pairs and showed that a significant portion of the variance in stages 2 and 4 sleep was genetically determined. Further studies performing PSA in 35 MZ and 14 DZ twins revealed significant genetic influences for duration of stage 3 and REM sleep, and significant genetic variance in spectral power extending from Δ to β frequencies.[45] More recently, EEG frequencies between 8 to 16 Hz have exhibited heritabilities as high as 96%, regardless of sleep need or intensity, potentially making this 1 of the most heritable traits in humans.[46] These data taken together suggest that EEG patterns represent a genetic fingerprint of sleep physiology in humans (**Table 2**).

Having established the heritability of sleep phenotypes, the question becomes whether or not individual sleep EEG phenotypes represent individual traits amenable to genetic investigation. Buckelmuller and colleagues[47] investigated intra-individual stability and interindividual variation in sleep EEG spectra across 4 baseline recordings of 8 healthy young men. They found substantial power spectral clustering within NREM EEG demonstrating low inter-individual similarity in contrast to high intra-individual similarity. All told this work supports traitlike characteristics of the sleep EEG and shows that this phenotype may be capable of facilitating identification of genes related to sleep physiology.

GENETIC STUDIES OF THE EEG IN ANIMAL MODELS

Animal models with readily observed EEG phenotypes provide a valuable resource to researchers interested in the genetic underpinnings of sleep neurophysiology. Like humans, sleep duration and organization are under strong genetic control in mice, with heritability estimates ranging between 40 to 60%.[48–52] Because the genetic contribution to spectral patterns of the sleep EEG in mice is much stronger than sleep amount and organization, mice are well suited to the genetic study of the EEG.[35,51–53]

Quantitative trait loci (QTL) are stretches of DNA that are closely linked to the genes that underlie the quantitative trait in question. Researchers have used large-scale QTL mapping techniques to isolate genes that underlie subtle differences in sleep architecture across inbred mouse strains.[54] Studies in inbred mice have shown that sleep distribution, amount, and sleep rebound are genetically controlled. It is estimated that half the variance observed for SWS and paradoxical sleep can be accounted for by genetic factors.[51,55] Indeed, QTL mapping of EEG Δ power (1–4 Hz) revealed a locus on chromosome 13 accounting for more than 50% of the genetic variance in this trait.[53] θ Oscillations, which vary in frequency across inbred mouse strains and predominate during paradoxical sleep and exploratory behavior, show minimal variation within a strain. θ Oscillation comparisons have been made between Balb/cByj mice, which have slow EEG θ frequencies, and c57bl/6J mice, which have fast EEG θ rhythms. Using QTL mapping, Tafti and colleagues[56] discovered that the short-chain acyl-coenzyme A dehydrogenase (Acads) gene was deficient in Balb/cByj mice, underlying the inherent slowing of their θ rhythms. QTL mapping in mice has also revealed a gene on chromosome 14, retinoic acid receptor β (*Rarb*), that contributes to the Δ frequency of 1 to 4 Hz in mice.[57] Retinoic acid receptors are believed to affect complex behaviors by influencing brain development and plasticity, possibly through effects on dopaminergic and cholinergic neurotransmission.[57–60] In this manner, the *Rarb* gene is believed to be important for modulating cortical synchrony during NREM sleep. These studies have shown that, in a mouse model, θ oscillations and SWS are regulated genetically and offer a means for further identification of factors underlying the sleep EEG, including SWS homeostasis. In addition, this work suggests the possibility that single genes may be found for quantitative EEG variants during sleep in humans.

Animal model knockouts have also been helpful in elucidating genetic aspects of the EEG, particularly regarding sleep neurochemistry and synaptic modulation. Acetylcholine is a part of the arousal system, critical for the waking EEG and REM sleep.[61] Mice lacking the nicotinic acetylcholine

Table 2
Twin studies of EEG during sleep

Study	Subjects (Years of Age)	EEG Parameters	Genetic Analysis	Results
Zung and Wilson,[38] 1966	4 MZ, 2 DZ; (8–19)	Sleep patterns	Visual inspection	MZ>DZ concordance
Webb and Campbell,[40] 1983	14 MZ, 14 DZ	PSG	Correlation	Sleep onset latency, awakening measures, stage changes, and REM amounts were correlated in MZ, but not DZ twins
Hori,[41,42] 1986, 1989	4 MZ, 3 DZ; (mean age 16)	PSG	Visual inspection, correlation	Sleep spindle density and periodicity, body movements, and REM cycle measures were correlated in MZ, but not DZ twins
Linkowski et al, 1989	14 MZ, 12 DZ; (16–35)	Sleep patterns; Δ sleep	Genetic variance analysis	Genetic influences on stage 2, 4, and Δ sleep
Linkowski et al,[44] 1991	11 MZ, 15 DZ	Sleep EEG	Genetic variance analysis	Genetic influence on stage 2 and 4
Ambrosius et al,[45] 2008	35 MZ (17–43), 14 DZ (18–26)	Sleep PSA; Δ, θ, α, β	Genetic variance analysis	Genetic influence on stages 3, 4, REM
De Gennaro et al,[46] 2008	10 MZ, 10 DZ, (24.6 ± 2.4)	Sleep PSA, 10–20 derivation	Genetic variance analysis	h^2 96% for 8–16 Hz frequencies

Abbreviations: DZ, dizygotic; h^2, heritability; MZ, monozygotic; PSA, power spectral analysis; PSG, polysomnogram; REM, rapid eye movement.
Adapted from van Beijsterveldt, van Baal GC. Twin and family studies of the human electroencephalogram: a review and meta-analysis. Biol Psychol 2002;61:114–7; with permission from Elsevier.

receptor β2 subunit gene show longer REM sleep episodes and reduced fragmentation of NREM sleep.[62] In contrast, mice lacking functional muscarinic acetylcholine M_3 receptors show decreased REM sleep and increased θ peak frequency in REM.[63] Although biogenic amines such as norepinephrine, dopamine, histamine, and serotonin have known wakefulness properties, little is known of their effect on the EEG. Serotonin is the exception, with clear evidence that it inhibits REM sleep and some studies showing that it may promote NREM sleep.[64–66] γ-Aminobutyric acid (GABA) is a major sleep-promoting neurotransmitter that inhibits wakefulness when released into the ventrolateral preoptic area. Knockout of various GABA subunits in mouse models has revealed variable effects on the EEG. GABA-A receptor a3 subunit knockout mice show reduced sleep spindle (10–15 Hz) activity.[67] Knockout of the GABA-A receptor d subunit has no effect on EEG patterns, although this has only been examined in the context of drug treatment.[68] The GABA-A receptor b3 subunit has been shown to influence REM sleep and EEG spectral phenomena associated with NREM sleep in mutant mice,[69] although these findings have been inconsistent.[70]

Adenosine is a multifunctional nucleoside that promotes sleep and reduces arousals as an inhibitory neurotransmitter and has been proposed as a homeostatic accumulator of sleep need.[71–73] During prolonged wakefulness, as ATP is degraded to ADP, AMP, and eventually adenosine, extracellular levels increase in sleep-promoting areas of the brain such as the basal forebrain and ventrolateral preoptic nucleus.[61] Therefore, the longer the wakeful period, the more adenosine accumulates, which signals a need for sleep, which serves to restore energy levels in the form of ATP. Mice expressing a dominant-negative soluble N-ethylmaleimide-sensitive factor attachment protein receptor (SNARE) protein that inhibits gliotransmission were found to have reduced cortical slow oscillations characteristic of NREM sleep, and also decreased sleep pressure following sleep deprivation.[74,75] This condition was postulated to be caused by decreased ATP release from astrocytes and subsequent attenuation of extracellular buildup of adenosine, which was believed to truncate the typical effects of adenosine on the A1 receptor; namely, suppression of synaptic transmission and promotion of SWA.[75]

Although the precise function of sleep remains a mystery, some researchers hypothesize that sleep may serve to downscale synaptic transmission, promoting neuronal efficiency and maintaining ratios of synaptic strength.[76] Differential expression studies of immediate early genes, genes that regulate synaptic strength, and genes that alter their expression based on sleep/wake state, such as NARP, Homer1a, c-Fos, and GluR3 AMPA receptor subunits, support this notion.[77–81] Knockout mice for c-Fos exhibit more wakefulness and reduced SWS, and GluR3-null animals show consistent reductions in Δ and θ frequency power in NREM sleep.[78,79] QTL analysis has identified the Homer1a gene as important to sleep homeostasis and Δ power.[80,81] This work as a whole shows an association between differential gene expression and aspects of the sleep EEG in NREM sleep. Further work with more precise synaptic phenotyping is necessary to establish synaptic downscaling as a definitive function of sleep.

Considering the importance of voltage-gated ion channels to maintenance of the membrane potential and generation of action potentials, one might think that genetic variability in ion channels and channel-regulating molecules would influence the EEG. Voltage-gated potassium channel mutations expressed in thalamocortical and GABAergic interneurons in the neocortex and hippocampus of mice have shown lower EEG power density in Δ and θ frequencies in NREM, and to a lesser extent REM, sleep, more prominent in frontal than occipital regions.[82–84] Potassium channel mutations have also been associated with decreased sleep spindle activity.[84] Mice lacking an N-type calcium channel α1b subunit show decreased power during NREM sleep and knockout mice for the α1G subunit of the T-type Ca^{++} channel exhibit decreased NREM cortical EEG oscillations, presumably because of the inability of thalamic relay neurons to go into bursting mode.[85,86] Confirmation of this finding with thalamus-specific knockout of this gene points to the importance of the thalamus in sleep EEG generation.[86] Similarly, mice lacking the SK2 channel (a thalamic nucleus reticularis dendrite–specific K^+ channel) show a threefold reduction in EEG Δ waves and reduced spindles along with substantially fragmented sleep.[87] Potassium channels such as these and T-type Ca^+ channels may couple, with further potential influences on sleep power spectra. This work confirms that voltage-gated ion channels exert substantial influence on aspects of the EEG in animal models, and provides intriguing possibilities for findings in humans.

Genes known to be involved in learning and memory, such as CREB, BDNF, and cGMP, have also been investigated for their potential role in the EEG phenotype.[3] CREB is a transcriptional regulator with influences on total and NREM sleep in mice, and mice lacking 1 of 2 CREB isoforms sleep longer and exhibit prolonged NREM sleep.[88,89] Brain-derived neurotrophic factor

(*BDNF*) is an important molecule for learning and memory. *BDNF* levels have been shown to increase in tandem with exploratory behavior, which in turn increases Δ power during sleep.[90] *BDNF* is a major target of *CREB*, so their influence on the sleep EEG may not be independent of one another.[3] Genetic manipulation of *cGMP*-dependent protein kinase influences quiescence in worms.[91] Mouse conditional brain knockouts of these kinases reduces REM sleep, increases sleep fragmentation, and are associated with increased Δ sleep rebound after sleep deprivation.[92]

Winrow and colleagues[93] took a comprehensive approach by performing a genome-wide scan for the various components of EEG-defined sleep by examining linkage between 2310 informative single nucleotide polymorphisms (SNPs) and 20 sleep-wake traits in 269 male mice from a genetically segregating population. They found 52 significant QTL, representing a minimum of 20 genomic loci, including REM and NREM power bands. Clustering of sleep phenotypes into trait-specific subnetworks revealed REM sleep as the most conserved subnetwork.[93] Taken together, this work reveals a complex genetic landscape underlying the sleep/wake EEG and emphasizes the need for a systems biology approach for elucidating the full extent of the genetic regulatory mechanisms of sleep neurophysiology.

In summary, use of QTL mapping and targeted genetic mutation in animals have improved our understanding of the neurogenetic aspects of sleep and the sleep EEG. Molecular genetic approaches in model organisms will continue to reveal the impact of genetic variation on sleep physiology. Tissue-specific gene expression will help clarify the sleep-related function of genes that are currently unknown. Neuron-specific alterations in voltage-gated ion channels will also allow a better understanding of sleep EEG phenotypes on both a macroscale and microscale. Gene expression profiling and targeted pharmacologic studies in well-defined subsets of neurons will also help elucidate the neuroanatomic molecular contributions to the EEG.

GENETIC STUDIES OF THE EEG IN HUMANS

Several genes, including adenosine deaminase (*ADA*), PERIOD3 (*PER3*), catechol-O-methyl-transferase (*COMT*), *5-HT3R*, and metabotropic glutamate receptor 8 (*GRM8*), have been identified as contributing to sleep EEG characteristics in humans (**Table 3**).[94,95] *ADA* is an enzyme involved in adenosine metabolism, and through this mechanism is felt to influence sleep phenotypes including the EEG. The *ADA* gene has several allelic variants

with wide-ranging effects on human physiology. One polymorphism in particular has been found with effects on the sleep EEG. Individuals heterozygous for the allelic variant of *ADA* carrying a G→A polymorphism at nucleotide 22 (*ADA* 22G/A genotype) exhibit roughly double the amount of stage 4 sleep, almost 30 minutes more SWS, and higher average absolute 0.5-Hz to 5.0-Hz EEG activity compared with subjects with the wild-type *ADA* G/G genotype.[94] It was shown that individuals with the G/A genotype exhibit 20% to 30% lower enzymatic activity in erythrocytes and leucocytes than individuals with the G/G genotype.[96] These results suggest that the *ADA* 22G→A polymorphism modulates both the duration of SWS as well as the intensity of sleep (**Fig. 4**).

The circadian system in mammals and invertebrates involves molecular feedback loops within cells that help to maintain a ~24-hour rhythm. (For further description of this, see the article by Zee in this issue.) The circadian clock is controlled by both positive and negative regulators. In mammals, positive regulators *BMAL1* and *NPAS2/CLOCK* drive the transcription of *PERIOD* (*PER*) and *CRYPTOCHROME* (*CRY*), which feed back to inhibit the transcription of the positive regulators mentioned earlier. Degradation of the negative regulators (*PER* and *CRY*) completes the cycle, allowing a new cycle to begin.[3] The *PER* gene (encompassing 3 homologs: *PER1*, *PER2*, and *PER3*) seems to be of particular importance to sleep architecture. The coding region of the *PER3* gene contains a variable-number tandem-repeat polymorphism (insertion of nucleotides 3031–3084) in which an 18–amino acid motif is repeated either 4 (*PER3*[4/4]) or 5 times (*PER3*[5/5]).[97] These repeat units contain a cluster of putative phosphorylation motifs.[98] Retrospective studies have shown that this polymorphism is associated with diurnal preference and delayed sleep-phase syndrome (DSPS).[98–100] Viola and colleagues[95] investigated the influence of this polymorphism on the sleep EEG by recruiting 24 healthy subjects based on their *PER3* genotype. The longer *PER3*[5/5] polymorphism was found to exert substantial influence on the sleep EEG. Specifically, SWS, EEG slow wave activity in NREM sleep, and θ and α activity during wakefulness and REM sleep were all increased in *PER3*[5/5] compared with *PER3*[4/4] individuals, supporting this polymorphism as an important marker of individual differences in sleep architecture or need. This work also suggests that *PER3*[5/5] individuals live with a higher sleep pressure than other genotypes.

Another gene associated with EEG phenotypes in humans is *5-HT3R*, a ligand-gated ion channel whose activation results in rapid neuronal

Table 3
Genetic variants associated with the human EEG

Gene	Genetic Variant	Chromosome	Putative Function	Influence on EEG
ADA	22G/A SNP rs11555565 rs73598374	20q13.11	Adenosine metabolism	Enhances deep sleep and slow wave activity during sleep
PER3[5/5]	Variable-number tandem repeat (54 bp) polymorphism (5 copies)	1p36.23	Encodes components of circadian rhythms of locomotion, activity, metabolism, and behavior	Enhances slow wave sleep, EEG slow wave activity in NREM sleep, θ and α activity during wakefulness and REM sleep
COMT	Val158Met SNP rs4680	22q11.2	Cortical dopamine metabolism	Increased power in the upper α range in wakefulness, REM, and NREM sleep
GRM8	14 SNPs: rs2402816 rs2299459 rs1158720 rs7797602 rs2402820 rs1074728 rs4731323 rs1361991 rs2299495 rs2299498 rs10256873 rs1361995 rs10487457 rs10487459	7q31.3-q32.1	Presynaptic autoreceptor controlling glutamate release	Event-related θ power
Serotonin receptor 5-HTR3B	3 SNPs: rs3782025 rs2276307 rs11606194	11q23.1	Subunit of the 5-HT3 serotonin receptor that is an excitatory ligand-gated ion channel	Resting EEG reduced α power

Abbreviations: ADA, adenosine deaminase; *COMT*, catechol-O-methyltransferase; *GRM8*, metabotropic glutamate receptor 8 gene; *PER3[5/5]*, period homolog 3[5/5].

depolarization. Three polymorphisms in this gene on chromosome 11 have been associated with lower EEG α power.[101] This finding has been confirmed in a linkage study in Plains Indians showing linkage of α EEG power to the same region on chromosome 11 where the *5-HT3R* gene is found.[101] One of the possible mechanisms by which *5-HT3R* might influence resting EEG is through the modulation of GABAergic interneurons located within the neocortex, hippocampus, and amygdala.

The human catechol-O-methyltransferase (*COMT*) gene is located on chromosome 22q11.2 and contains a functional SNP that alters the amino acid sequence of the membrane-bound *COMT* protein at codon 158 from valine (*Val*) to methionine

(*Met*).[102] Individuals who are homozygous for the *Val* allele show more *COMT* protein in postmortem brain tissue than individuals with 2 *Met* alleles.[103] Moreover, *Val/Val* genotype subjects show threefold to fourfold higher *COMT* activity and, presumably, lower dopaminergic signaling in the prefrontal cortex than do *Met/Met* genotype subjects.[103,104] Recently, it has been shown that the Val158Met polymorphism predicts stable and frequency-specific, interindividual variation in brain α oscillations. α Peak frequency in wakefulness was 1.4 Hz slower in Val/Val genotype than in Met/Met genotype. Moreover, Val/Val allele carriers exhibited less activity at 11 to 13 Hz than Met/Met homozygotes in wakefulness, REM, and non-REM sleep.[105] This same polymorphism is strongly associated with Δ and θ activity in

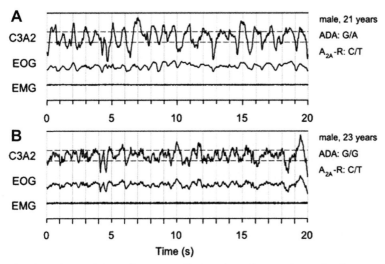

Fig. 4. Higher amplitude and prevalence of EEG Δ oscillations in a 20-second sample of stage-4 sleep in an individual with the G/A ADA genotype (*A*) than in an individual with the G/G genotype (*B*). C3A2, EEG derivation; EOG, bipolar electro-oculogram; EMG, submental electromyogram. Horizontal dashed lines below and above the EEG trace indicate 75 μV. (*Reproduced from* Retey JV, Adam M, Honegger E, et al. A functional genetic variation of adenosine deaminase affects the duration and intensity of deep sleep in humans. Proc Natl Acad Sci U S A 2005;102(43):15678; with permission from Proceedings of the National Academy of Sciences USA, Copyright 2005.)

patients with schizophrenia.[106] This work suggests that fluctuations in cortical dopamine levels exert broad influence on resting brain states and the EEG power spectra in humans.

Genome-wide linkage scans of event-related θ band power have shown significant linkage (peak logarithm of the odds = 3.5) to chromosome 7q31.3-q32.1.[107,108] Using this information, Chen and colleagues[109] focused on genetic variation in the metabotropic glutamate receptor 8 gene (*GRM8*), primarily based on proximity of this gene to this chromosomal region. They found evidence for 14 *GRM8* SNPs associated with θ band power. Electrophysiologic and morphologic studies suggested that the *mGluR8* receptor is localized at the presynaptic grid of glutamate synapses, and it functions as a presynaptic autoreceptor controlling glutamate release from the lateral perforant path terminals in the dentate gyrus.[110] This work suggests that neuronal oscillations may represent endophenotypes of glutamate neurotransmission, or, alternatively, that glutamatergic neurotransmission underlies human variability in EEG signals.

Many studies assessing genetic variation in the human EEG focus on highly selected populations. These studies assess SNPs in specific genes, based on biologic plausibility and results from previous animal studies. To truly understand the influence of genetic variation on the sleep EEG, large population-based cohorts with dense

genotyping and extensive EEG phenotyping are needed. Some of these studies are underway, and their results are eagerly anticipated because they will likely reveal novel pathways involved with sleep generation and maintenance and possibly provide targets for drug development intended to improve sleep quality.

SUMMARY

Despite all that has been learned regarding sleep and sleep physiology, the physiologic nature of sleep remains elusive. Some of the more accepted hypotheses include maintenance of cellular, immune, and metabolic function, synaptic downscaling, and memory consolidation.[3] Genetic investigations may help answer some of these questions, but only if the phenotype in question is rigorously defined. The EEG is well suited for this task, because it is meaningfully associated with sleep, stable over time, and under significant genetic control. From an objective standpoint, few phenotypes in sleep are more precise than the EEG.

Future studies assessing the genetics of the EEG can take several approaches to advance the field. Genomic technologies can be leveraged to assess genome-wide association of SNPs and copy number variation with various EEG phenotypes. Genetic manipulation of candidate genes based on hypothesized sleep functions can be assessed for influence on EEG phenotypes. The EEG itself can be manipulated and the epigenetic ramifications can be measured, including gene expression levels. High-density EEG and ultraslow direct current EEG provide compelling avenues to further expand and specify the EEG phenotype for genetic studies. Currently there is no evidence that a single gene, or subset of genes, acting in a specific set of neurons is responsible for sleep, therefore it is likely that future studies will complicate rather than simplify our understanding of the genetics of the EEG. For this reason, network and systems biologic approaches assessing interrelationships of various genetic variants and assessment of their combined influence on EEG phenotypes may be necessary to unravel the polygenetic nature of this complicated phenotype.

ACKNOWLEDGMENTS

I would like to thank Roseanne Armitage for providing a figure for this manuscript.

REFERENCES

1. Swartz BE, Goldensohn ES. Timeline of the history of EEG and associated fields. Electroencephalogr Clin Neurophysiol 1998;106:173–6.
2. Kandel ER, Schwartz JH, Jessell TM. Principles of Neural Science. 4th edition. New York: McGraw-Hill; 2000.
3. Crocker A, Sehgal A. Genetic analysis of sleep. Genes Dev 2010;24:1220–35.
4. Tobler I, Borbely AA. Sleep EEG in the rat as a function of prior waking. Electroencephalogr Clin Neurophysiol 1986;64:74–6.
5. Boomsma D, Busjahn A, Peltonen L. Classical twin studies and beyond. Nat Rev Genet 2002;3: 872–82.
6. Davis H, Davis P. Action potentials of the brain. Arch Neurol 1936;36:1214–24.
7. Dieker H. Studies on the genetics of particularly regular high alpha-waves in human EEG. Humangenetik 1967;4:189–216 [in German].
8. Gottlober AB. The inheritance of brain potentials. J Exp Psychol 1938;22:193–200.
9. Hueschert D. EEG-untersuchungen an eineiigen zwillungen in hoheren lebensalter. Z Mensch Vereb Konstitutionsl 1963;37:128–72.
10. Juel-Nielsen N, Harvald B. The electroencephalogram in uniovular twins brought up apart. Acta Genet Stat Med 1958;8:57–64.
11. Lennox W, Gibbs E, Gibbs F. The brain-wave pattern an hereditary trait: evidence from 74 'normal' pairs of twins. J Hered 1945;36:233–43.
12. Raney E. Brain potentials and lateral dominance in identical twins. J Exp Psychol 1939;24:21–39.
13. Vogel F. Uber die erblichkeit des normalen Elektroenzephalogramms: vergleichende Untersuchungen an ein- und zweieigen Zwillingen. Stuttgart (Germany): Thieme; 1958.
14. Vogel F. Of the genetic basis of slow occipital beta waves in human EEG. Humangenetik 1966;2: 238–45 [in German].
15. Vogel F. Of the genetic basis of fronto-precentral beta wave groups in human EEG. Humangenetik 1966;2:227–37 [in German].
16. Young JP, Lader MH, Fenton GW. A twin study of the genetic influences on the electroencephalogram. J Med Genet 1972;9:13–6.
17. Hume W, editor. Physiological measures in twins. Oxford (NY): Pergamon; 1983.
18. Stassen HH, Lykken DT, Propping P, et al. Genetic determination of the human EEG. Survey of recent results on twins reared together and apart. Hum Genet 1988;80:165–76.
19. Gao Y, Tuvblad C, Raine A, et al. Genetic and environmental influences on frontal EEG asymmetry and alpha power in 9-10-year-old twins. Psychophysiology 2009;46:787–96.
20. Steinlein O, Anokhin A, Yping M, et al. Localization of a gene for the human low-voltage EEG on 20q and genetic heterogeneity. Genomics 1992;12:69–73.
21. Lykken DT, Tellegen A, Iacono WG. EEG spectra on twins: evidence for a neglected mechanism of genetic determination. Physiol Psychol 1982;10: 60–5.
22. Lykken DT, Tellegen A, Thorkelson K. Genetic determination of EEG frequency spectra. Biol Psychol 1974;1:245–59.
23. Meshkova T, Ravich-Shcherbo I, editors. Influence of the genotype on the determination of individual features of the human EEG at rest. Berlin: VEB Deutscher Verlag der Wissenshaft; 1982.
24. Propping P. Genetic control of ethanol action on the central nervous system. An EEG study in twins. Hum Genet 1977;35:309–34.
25. Whitton JL, Elgie SM, Kugel H, et al. Genetic dependence of the electroencephalogram bispectrum. Electroencephalogr Clin Neurophysiol 1985; 60:293–8.
26. McGuire KA, Katsanis J, Iacono WG, et al. Genetic influences on the spontaneous EEG: and examination of 15-year-old and 17-year-old twins. Dev Neuropsychol 1998;14:7–18.
27. Christian JC, Morzorati S, Norton JA Jr, et al. Genetic analysis of the resting electroencephalographic power spectrum in human twins. Psychophysiology 1996;33:584–91.
28. Van Baal GC, De Geus EJ, Boomsma DI. Genetic architecture of EEG power spectra in early life. Electroencephalogr Clin Neurophysiol 1996;98:502–14.
29. van Beijsterveldt CE, Molenaar PC, de Geus EJ, et al. Heritability of human brain functioning as

assessed by electroencephalography. Am J Hum Genet 1996;58:562–73.

30. van Beijsterveldt CE, Molenaar PC, de Geus EJ, et al. Genetic and environmental influences on EEG coherence. Behav Genet 1998;28:443–53.

31. van Baal GC, de Geus EJ, Boomsma DI. Genetic influences on EEG coherence in 5-year-old twins. Behav Genet 1998;28:9–19.

32. van Baal GC, Boomsma DI, de Geus EJ. Longitudinal genetic analysis of EEG coherence in young twins. Behav Genet 2001;31:637–51.

33. Posthuma D, Neale MC, Boomsma DI, et al. Are smarter brains running faster? Heritability of alpha peak frequency, IQ, and their interrelation. Behav Genet 2001;31:567–79.

34. van Beijsterveldt CE, van Baal GC. Twin and family studies of the human electroencephalogram: a review and a meta-analysis. Biol Psychol 2002; 61:111–38.

35. Dauvilliers Y, Maret S, Tafti M. Genetics of normal and pathological sleep in humans. Sleep Med Rev 2005;9:91–100.

36. de Castro JM. The influence of heredity on self-reported sleep patterns in free-living humans. Physiol Behav 2002;76:479–86.

37. Heath AC, Kendler KS, Eaves LJ, et al. Evidence for genetic influences on sleep disturbance and sleep pattern in twins. Sleep 1990;13:318–35.

38. Zung WW, Wilson WP. Sleep and dream patterns in twins. Markov analysis of a genetic trait. Recent Adv Biol Psychiatry 1966;9:119–30.

39. Gould J, Austin F, Cook P. A genetic analysis of sleep stage organization in newborn twins. Sleep Res 1978;7:132.

40. Webb WB, Campbell SS. Relationships in sleep characteristics of identical and fraternal twins. Arch Gen Psychiatry 1983;40:1093–5.

41. Hori A. Sleep characteristics in twins. Jpn J Psychiatry Neurol 1986;40:35–46.

42. Hori A, Kazukawa S, Endo M, et al. Sleep spindles in twins. Clin Electroencephalogr 1989;20:121–7.

43. Linkowski P. EEG sleep patterns in twins. J Sleep Res 1999;8(Suppl 1):11–3.

44. Linkowski P, Kerkhofs M, Hauspie R, et al. Genetic determinants of EEG sleep: a study in twins living apart. Electroencephalogr Clin Neurophysiol 1991; 79:114–8.

45. Ambrosius U, Lietzenmaier S, Wehrle R, et al. Heritability of sleep electroencephalogram. Biol Psychiatry 2008;64:344–8.

46. De Gennaro L, Marzano C, Fratello F, et al. The electroencephalographic fingerprint of sleep is genetically determined: a twin study. Ann Neurol 2008;64:455–60.

47. Buckelmuller J, Landolt HP, Stassen HH, et al. Trait-like individual differences in the human sleep electroencephalogram. Neuroscience 2006;138:351–6.

48. Valatx JL, Bugat R, Jouvet M. Genetic studies of sleep in mice. Nature 1972;238:226–7.

49. Tafti M, Franken P, Kitahama K, et al. Localization of candidate genomic regions influencing paradoxical sleep in mice. Neuroreport 1997;8:3755–8.

50. Tafti M, Chollet D, Valatx JL, et al. Quantitative trait loci approach to the genetics of sleep in recombinant inbred mice. J Sleep Res 1999;8(Suppl 1): 37–43.

51. Franken P, Malafosse A, Tafti M. Genetic determinants of sleep regulation in inbred mice. Sleep 1999;22:155–69.

52. Franken P, Malafosse A, Tafti M. Genetic variation in EEG activity during sleep in inbred mice. Am J Physiol 1998;275:R1127–37.

53. Franken P, Chollet D, Tafti M. The homeostatic regulation of sleep need is under genetic control. J Neurosci 2001;21:2610–21.

54. O'Hara BF, Ding J, Bernat RL, et al. Genomic and proteomic approaches towards an understanding of sleep. CNS Neurol Disord Drug Targets 2007;6: 71–81.

55. Tafti M, Franken P. Invited review: genetic dissection of sleep. J Appl Physiol 2002;92:1339–47.

56. Tafti M, Petit B, Chollet D, et al. Deficiency in short-chain fatty acid beta-oxidation affects theta oscillations during sleep. Nat Genet 2003;34:320–5.

57. Maret S, Franken P, Dauvilliers Y, et al. Retinoic acid signaling affects cortical synchrony during sleep. Science 2005;310:111–3.

58. Krezel W, Ghyselinck N, Samad TA, et al. Impaired locomotion and dopamine signaling in retinoid receptor mutant mice. Science 1998;279:863–7.

59. Farooqui SM. Induction of adenylate cyclase sensitive dopamine D2-receptors in retinoic acid induced differentiated human neuroblastoma SHSY-5Y cells. Life Sci 1994;55:1887–93.

60. Pedersen WA, Berse B, Schuler U, et al. All-trans- and 9-cis-retinoic acid enhance the cholinergic properties of a murine septal cell line: evidence that the effects are mediated by activation of retinoic acid receptor-alpha. J Neurochem 1995;65:50–8.

61. Saper CB, Scammell TE, Lu J. Hypothalamic regulation of sleep and circadian rhythms. Nature 2005; 437:1257–63.

62. Lena C, Popa D, Grailhe R, et al. Beta2-containing nicotinic receptors contribute to the organization of sleep and regulate putative micro-arousals in mice. J Neurosci 2004;24:5711–8.

63. Goutagny R, Comte JC, Salvert D, et al. Paradoxical sleep in mice lacking M3 and M2/M4 muscarinic receptors. Neuropsychobiology 2005;52: 140–6.

64. Boutrel B, Franc B, Hen R, et al. Key role of 5-HT1B receptors in the regulation of paradoxical sleep as evidenced in 5-HT1B knock-out mice. J Neurosci 1999;19:3204–12.

65. Boutrel B, Monaca C, Hen R, et al. Involvement of 5-HT1A receptors in homeostatic and stress-induced adaptive regulations of paradoxical sleep: studies in 5-HT1A knock-out mice. J Neurosci 2002;22:4686–92.

66. Jouvet M. Insomnia and decrease of cerebral 5-hydroxytryptamine after destruction of the raphe system in the cat. Adv Pharmacol 1968;6: 265–79.

67. Winsky-Sommerer R, Knapman A, Fedele DE, et al. Normal sleep homeostasis and lack of epilepsy phenotype in GABA A receptor alpha3 subunit-knockout mice. Neuroscience 2008;154: 595–605.

68. Winsky-Sommerer R, Vyazovskiy VV, Homanics GE, et al. The EEG effects of THIP (Gaboxadol) on sleep and waking are mediated by the GABA(A) a3 subunit-containing receptors. Eur J Neurosci 2007; 25:1893–9.

69. Wisor JP, DeLorey TM, Homanics GE, et al. Sleep states and sleep electroencephalographic spectral power in mice lacking the beta 3 subunit of the GABA(A) receptor. Brain Res 2002;955:221–8.

70. Laposky AD, Homanics GE, Basile A, et al. Deletion of the GABA(A) receptor beta 3 subunit eliminates the hypnotic actions of oleamide in mice. Neuroreport 2001;12:4143–7.

71. Benington JH, Heller HC. Restoration of brain energy metabolism as the function of sleep. Prog Neurobiol 1995;45:347–60.

72. Radulovacki M, Virus RM, Djuricic-Nedelson M, et al. Adenosine analogs and sleep in rats. J Pharmacol Exp Ther 1984;228:268–74.

73. Strecker RE, Morairty S, Thakkar MM, et al. Adenosinergic modulation of basal forebrain and preoptic/anterior hypothalamic neuronal activity in the control of behavioral state. Behav Brain Res 2000;115:183–204.

74. Halassa MM, Florian C, Fellin T, et al. Astrocytic modulation of sleep homeostasis and cognitive consequences of sleep loss. Neuron 2009;61: 213–9.

75. Fellin T, Halassa MM, Terunuma M, et al. Endogenous nonneuronal modulators of synaptic transmission control cortical slow oscillations in vivo. Proc Natl Acad Sci U S A 2009;106:15037–42.

76. Tononi G, Cirelli C. Sleep function and synaptic homeostasis. Sleep Med Rev 2006;10:49–62.

77. Cirelli C, LaVaute TM, Tononi G. Sleep and wakefulness modulate gene expression in Drosophila. J Neurochem 2005;94:1411–9.

78. Shiromani PJ, Basheer R, Thakkar J, et al. Sleep and wakefulness in c-fos and fos B gene knockout mice. Brain Res Mol Brain Res 2000;80:75–87.

79. Steenland HW, Kim SS, Zhuo M. GluR3 subunit regulates sleep, breathing and seizure generation. Eur J Neurosci 2008;27:1166–73.

80. Mackiewicz M, Paigen B, Naidoo N, et al. Analysis of the QTL for sleep homeostasis in mice: Homer1a is a likely candidate. Physiol Genomics 2008;33: 91–9.

81. Maret S, Dorsaz S, Gurcel L, et al. Homer1a is a core brain molecular correlate of sleep loss. Proc Natl Acad Sci U S A 2007;104:20090–5.

82. Vyazovskiy VV, Deboer T, Rudy B, et al. Sleep EEG in mice that are deficient in the potassium channel subunit K.v.3.2. Brain Res 2002;947:204–11.

83. Douglas CL, Vyazovskiy V, Southard T, et al. Sleep in Kcna2 knockout mice. BMC Biol 2007;5:42.

84. Espinosa F, Torres-Vega MA, Marks GA, et al. Ablation of Kv3.1 and Kv3.3 potassium channels disrupts thalamocortical oscillations in vitro and in vivo. J Neurosci 2008;28:5570–81.

85. Lee J, Kim D, Shin HS. Lack of delta waves and sleep disturbances during non-rapid eye movement sleep in mice lacking alpha1G-subunit of T-type calcium channels. Proc Natl Acad Sci U S A 2004;101:18195–9.

86. Anderson MP, Mochizuki T, Xie J, et al. Thalamic Cav3.1 T-type Ca2+ channel plays a crucial role in stabilizing sleep. Proc Natl Acad Sci U S A 2005;102:1743–8.

87. Cueni L, Canepari M, Lujan R, et al. T-type Ca2+ channels, SK2 channels and SERCAs gate sleep-related oscillations in thalamic dendrites. Nat Neurosci 2008;11:683–92.

88. Graves L, Dalvi A, Lucki I, et al. Behavioral analysis of CREB alphadelta mutation on a B6/129 F1 hybrid background. Hippocampus 2002;12:18–26.

89. Graves LA, Hellman K, Veasey S, et al. Genetic evidence for a role of CREB in sustained cortical arousal. J Neurophysiol 2003;90:1152–9.

90. Huber R, Tononi G, Cirelli C. Exploratory behavior, cortical BDNF expression, and sleep homeostasis. Sleep 2007;30:129–39.

91. Raizen DM, Zimmerman JE, Maycock MH, et al. Lethargus is a Caenorhabditis elegans sleep-like state. Nature 2008;451:569–72.

92. Langmesser S, Franken P, Feil S, et al. cGMP-dependent protein kinase type I is implicated in the regulation of the timing and quality of sleep and wakefulness. PLoS One 2009;4:e4238.

93. Winrow CJ, Williams DL, Kasarskis A, et al. Uncovering the genetic landscape for multiple sleep-wake traits. PLoS One 2009;4:e5161.

94. Retey JV, Adam M, Honegger E, et al. A functional genetic variation of adenosine deaminase affects the duration and intensity of deep sleep in humans. Proc Natl Acad Sci U S A 2005;102:15676–81.

95. Viola AU, Archer SN, James LM, et al. PER3 polymorphism predicts sleep structure and waking performance. Curr Biol 2007;17:613–8.

96. Battistuzzi G, Iudicone P, Santolamazza P, et al. Activity of adenosine deaminase allelic forms in

intact erythrocytes and in lymphocytes. Ann Hum Genet 1981;45:15–9.

97. Ebisawa T, Uchiyama M, Kajimura N, et al. Association of structural polymorphisms in the human period3 gene with delayed sleep phase syndrome. EMBO Rep 2001;2:342–6.

98. Archer SN, Robilliard DL, Skene DJ, et al. A length polymorphism in the circadian clock gene Per3 is linked to delayed sleep phase syndrome and extreme diurnal preference. Sleep 2003;26:413–5.

99. Jones KH, Ellis J, von Schantz M, et al. Age-related change in the association between a polymorphism in the PER3 gene and preferred timing of sleep and waking activities. J Sleep Res 2007;16:12–6.

100. Pereira DS, Tufik S, Louzada FM, et al. Association of the length polymorphism in the human Per3 gene with the delayed sleep-phase syndrome: does latitude have an influence upon it? Sleep 2005;28:29–32.

101. Ducci F, Enoch MA, Yuan Q, et al. HTR3B is associated with alcoholism with antisocial behavior and alpha EEG power–an intermediate phenotype for alcoholism and co-morbid behaviors. Alcohol 2009;43:73–84.

102. Bodenmann S, Xu S, Luhmann UF, et al. Pharmacogenetics of modafinil after sleep loss: catechol-O-methyltransferase genotype modulates waking functions but not recovery sleep. Clin Pharmacol Ther 2009;85:296–304.

103. Chen J, Lipska BK, Halim N, et al. Functional analysis of genetic variation in catechol-O-methyltransferase (COMT): effects on mRNA, protein, and enzyme activity in postmortem human brain. Am J Hum Genet 2004;75:807–21.

104. Akil M, Kolachana BS, Rothmond DA, et al. Catechol-O-methyltransferase genotype and dopamine regulation in the human brain. J Neurosci 2003;23: 2008–13.

105. Bodenmann S, Rusterholz T, Durr R, et al. The functional Val158Met polymorphism of COMT predicts interindividual differences in brain alpha oscillations in young men. J Neurosci 2009;29:10855–62.

106. Venables NC, Bernat EM, Sponheim SR. Genetic and disorder-specific aspects of resting state EEG abnormalities in schizophrenia. Schizophr Bull 2009;35:826–39.

107. Jones KA, Porjesz B, Almasy L, et al. Linkage and linkage disequilibrium of evoked EEG oscillations with CHRM2 receptor gene polymorphisms: implications for human brain dynamics and cognition. Int J Psychophysiol 2004;53:75–90.

108. Jones KA, Porjesz B, Almasy L, et al. A cholinergic receptor gene (CHRM2) affects event-related oscillations. Behav Genet 2006;36:627–39.

109. Chen AC, Tang Y, Rangaswamy M, et al. Association of single nucleotide polymorphisms in a glutamate receptor gene (GRM8) with theta power of event-related oscillations and alcohol dependence. Am J Med Genet B Neuropsychiatr Genet 2009; 150B:359–68.

110. Shigemoto R, Kinoshita A, Wada E, et al. Differential presynaptic localization of metabotropic glutamate receptor subtypes in the rat hippocampus. J Neurosci 1997;17:7503–22.

Genetics of Sleep Timing, Duration, and Homeostasis in Humans

Namni Goel, PhD

KEYWORDS
- Genetics • Sleep duration • Sleep homeostasis
- Sleep deprivation • Circadian timing • Individual differences

Both sleep and wakefulness are modulated by an endogenous biological clock located in the supra-chiasmatic nuclei (SCN) of the anterior hypothalamus. Beyond driving the body to fall asleep and to wake up, the biological clock also modulates waking behavior, as reflected in sleepiness and cognitive performance, generating circadian rhythmicity in almost all neurobehavioral variables investigated to date.[1,2] Theoretical conceptualizations of the daily temporal modulation of sleep and wakefulness (and to a lesser extent the modulation of waking cognitive functions) have been instantiated in the two-process mathematical model of sleep regulation[3,4] and its mathematical variants.[5] The two-process model of sleep regulation has been applied to the temporal profiles of sleep[4,6] and wakefulness.[7] The model consists of a sleep homeostatic process (S) and a circadian process (C), which interact to determine the timing of sleep onset and offset, as well as the stability of waking neurocognitive functions.[1,2,8] The homeostatic process represents the drive for sleep that increases during wakefulness (as can be observed when wakefulness is maintained beyond habitual bedtime into the night and subsequent day) and

decreases during sleep (which represents recuperation obtained from sleep). When this homeostatic drive increases above a certain threshold, sleep is triggered; when it decreases below a different threshold, wakefulness is invoked. The circadian process represents daily oscillatory modulation of these threshold levels. It has been suggested that the circadian system actively promotes wakefulness more than sleep,[9] although this hypothesis is not presently universally accepted. The circadian drive for wakefulness may be experienced as spontaneously enhanced alertness in the early evening even after a sleepless night. Sleep deprivation, however, can elevate homeostatic pressure to the point that waking cognitive functions are degraded even at the time of the peak circadian drive for wakefulness.[10] There are robust individual differences in both the sleep homeostatic and circadian processes, pointing to genetic underpinnings.

This review begins with a discussion of the genetic basis of circadian rhythms and the timing of sleep. It next briefly discusses the genetic basis of sleep in healthy adults, including observed individual variability in sleep parameters. Next, it

The writing of this article was supported by National Space Biomedical Research Institute through NASA NCC 9-58, NIH NR004281 and CTRC UL1RR024134, and by a grant from the Institute for Translational Medicine and Therapeutics' (ITMAT) Transdisciplinary Program in Translational Medicine and Therapeutics. The project described was supported in part by Grant Number UL1RR024134 from the National Center for Research Resources. The content is solely the responsibility of the authors and does not necessarily represent the official views of the National Center for Research Resources or the National Institutes of Health.
The author has nothing to disclose.

Division of Sleep and Chronobiology, Unit for Experimental Psychiatry, Department of Psychiatry, University of Pennsylvania School of Medicine, 1013 Blockley Hall, 423 Guardian Drive, Philadelphia, PA 19104-6021, USA
E-mail address: goel@mail.med.upenn.edu

Sleep Med Clin 6 (2011) 171–182
doi:10.1016/j.jsmc.2011.03.004
1556-407X/11/$ – see front matter © 2011 Elsevier Inc. All rights reserved.

discusses individual differences in the context of the total absence of sleep and the restriction of sleep as phenotypes, and recent studies using candidate gene approaches to identify genes that may relate to such responses. Finally, future areas of research are discussed.

GENETICS OF INDIVIDUAL DIFFERENCES IN CIRCADIAN RHYTHMS AND THE TIMING OF SLEEP

There are genetic underpinnings of individual differences in the circadian system, which are important for the timing of sleep. Morningness-eveningness (ie, the tendency to be an early "lark" or a late "owl") is perhaps the most frequently used measure of interindividual variation in circadian rhythmicity. Morning-type and evening-type individuals differ endogenously in the circadian phase of their biological clocks.[11,12] Self-report measures, such as the Horne-Östberg morningness-eveningness questionnaire (MEQ[13]) and its variants (eg, Ref.[14]), and more recent scales such as the Munich ChronoType Questionnaire,[15,16] which differentiates timing of activities on workdays versus free days, are the most commonly used measures of circadian phase preference, mainly because of their convenience and cost effectiveness.

Age influences morningness-eveningness, as shown in laboratory studies[17] and in more naturalistic population-based settings (see for reviews Refs.[16,18]). In addition, gender also affects morningness-eveningness, whereby women show a greater skew toward morningness than men.[16,19,20] This circadian phase preference difference is an enduring trait, with a significant genetic basis.[21–23] Thus, chronotype represents a circadian rhythmicity phenotype in humans.[24]

The genetic basis of morningness-eveningness in the general population has been investigated in several core circadian genes, with mixed results.[25] For example, the 3111C allele of the CLOCK gene 5'-untranslated region (5'-UTR) has been associated with eveningness and delayed sleep timing in some studies,[26,27] but not others.[28–30] Similarly, the variable number tandem repeat (VNTR) polymorphism in PERIOD3 (PER3), another core clock gene, has been linked to diurnal preference, but not uniformly so.[31–36] Both the 111G polymorphism in the 5'-UTR of PERIOD2 (PER2) and the T2434C polymorphism of PERIOD1 (PER1) also have been associated with morning preference.[37,38] Because morningness-eveningness represents a continuum, this trait is likely polygenic, influenced by several genes, each contributing to the determination of circadian phase preference. Thus, further

studies investigating other clock genes, as well as replication of the PER and CLOCK findings, are needed to establish precisely the molecular genetic components of behavioral circadian phase preference.

Individual differences in morningness-eveningness (chronotype) can manifest into extreme cases classified as primary circadian rhythm sleep disorders (CRSDs), with altered phase relationships of the biological clock to the light-dark cycle, including alterations in sleep timing.[39,40] Thus, extreme eveningness is believed to result in CRSD, delayed sleep phase type (typically referred to as a disorder and abbreviated as DSPD[40]), whereas extreme morningness can manifest as CRSD, advanced sleep phase type[39] (typically referred to as a disorder and abbreviated as ASPD[40]). The extent to which these phase-displacement disorders reflect differences in endogenous circadian period, entrainment, amplitude, coupling, and other aspects of clock neurobiology has received recent attention.

The genetic basis of DSPD and ASPD has been investigated in recent years, with both disorders having links to core clock genes.[25] DSPD, the most common circadian rhythm sleep disorder in the general population, is characterized by an inability to fall asleep at the desired and "normal" time of day; the average onset of sleep in DSPD occurs in the early morning (3 AM–6 AM), and the average wake-up time occurs in the late morning to early afternoon (11 AM–2 PM).[40] DSPD also may be characterized by a longer than normal tau (25.38 hours).[41] The VNTR polymorphism in PER3 is associated with DSPD in large sample studies,[31,32,34] and the 3111C allele of the CLOCK gene 5'-UTR region also has been related to DSPD.[26] A specific haplotype of PER3, which includes the polymorphism G647, is also associated positively with DSPD,[34] while the N408 allele of casein kinase I epsilon (CK1ε) may protect against the development of DSPD.[42]

ASPD is a rare disorder characterized by 3- to 4-hour advanced sleep onsets and wake times relative to desired, normal times.[40,43] It may be characterized by a shorter than normal tau (23.3 hours).[44] In one study, ASPD was associated with a mutation in PER2,[45] although this mutation is not found in all families with this disorder.[46] Another study has implicated mutations in casein kinase I delta (CK1δ) in ASPD.[47] Future studies on additional core clock genes are needed to determine other mutations which may underlie this disorder.

Morningness-eveningness and differences in circadian phase preference are reflected in the diurnal course of neurobehavioral variables (as reviewed in Ref.[48])—some people perform consistently better in the morning, whereas others are more alert and perform better in the evening. How genetic variants underlying morningness-eveningness and disorders of chronotype affect performance and alertness under normal and sleep-deprived conditions remains a new field of investigation. Recent studies[35,36,49] have shown that the longer, 5-repeat allele of the VNTR polymorphism in PER3, a clock gene linked to diurnal preference and DSPD, may be associated with higher sleep propensity both at baseline and after total sleep deprivation (TSD), and worse cognitive performance following TSD and higher sleep propensity during chronic partial sleep deprivation (PSD) (see later discussion for more detail of these studies). The role of other clock gene polymorphisms such as the 3111C allele of the CLOCK gene in response to TSD and to chronic PSD remain unknown and are worthy of investigation.

Six core clock genes (PER1, PER2, PER3, CLOCK, CK1δ, CK1ε) have thus far been associated with interindividual differences in diurnal preference or its extreme variants. This active area of research has promising implications for objectively detecting individual differences in circadian disorders, and determining situations and lifestyles that adversely affect the timing of sleep and sleep homeostasis.

GENETICS OF SLEEP

Sleep is a highly complex trait that involves many genes and their interactions with environmental factors. In humans, research dating back to as early as the 1930s employing twins has indicated a strong genetic basis underlying the regulation of normal sleep, including sleep duration, sleep onset, sleep quality, and sleep homeostasis (reviewed in Refs.[50–52]). In addition, in 2008, two studies in normal sleepers found strong heritability of the sleep electroencephalography (EEG) power spectrum, underscoring prior studies indicating that while the sleep EEG is consistent across nights in the same individual, it differs among individuals.[53,54] The genetic nature of the sleep EEG is also observed across a variety of frequencies indicating trait-like features.[55–60] Moreover, waking EEG patterns are also highly heritable (reviewed in Ref.[52]). Of note, familial linkage studies on EEG traits are currently lacking (reviewed in Refs.[50,61]).

More recently, candidate gene studies have investigated the role of specific genes in the regulation of sleep. For example, a point mutation in the DEC2 gene, believed to function in the circadian clock as a repressor of Clock/Bmal1, is associated with a short sleep duration phenotype (average 6.25 hours vs 8.06 hours of self-reported sleep) that is characterized by an earlier non-workday habitual sleep offset time, with normal onset time, in 2 adults.[62] Moreover, the insertion of this point mutation into mice also decreased sleep time without affecting tau. Future studies should determine the role of this DEC2 mutation in individuals undergoing sleep deprivation and in studies using EEG and slow-wave activity (SWA) physiologic sleep assessments for sleep duration, sleep homeostasis, and other related variables. By contrast, a recent study found that a polymorphism within intron 8 of the dopamine transporter 1 (DAT1) gene failed to correlate with the interindividual variability of basal polysomnographic sleep architecture, including slow-wave sleep latency, rapid eye movement (REM) sleep latency, sleep efficiency, and sleep stage percentages (stages 1, 2, slow-wave sleep, and REM) in a group of unrelated healthy men.[63]

CANDIDATE GENE STUDIES OF SLEEP DEPRIVATION

Beyond these studies, which assess habitual sleep or one night of baseline sleep, candidate gene studies have been used to study basal (fully rested) sleep and responses to sleep loss. This approach was motivated by the results of studies that indicated that there are stable phenotypic individual differences in response to sleep deprivation.

Subjects undergoing TSD display differential vulnerability to sleep loss, demonstrating robust interindividual differences in response to the same laboratory conditions, as measured by various physiologic and subjective sleep measures and neurobehavioral tasks sensitive to sleep loss.[59,64–68] Approximately one-third of healthy adults are highly vulnerable to the neurobehavioral effects of sleep deprivation, another third are vulnerable, and the remaining third are much less vulnerable. These stable (phenotypic) differences in neurobehavioral responses to sleep deprivation are not reliably accounted for thus far by demographic factors (eg, age, sex, IQ), by baseline functioning, by various aspects of habitual sleep timing, by circadian chronotype, or by any other investigated factor.[10,64,69,70]

Such differential vulnerability extends to chronic PSD—a condition associated with a wide range of serious health consequences and experienced by millions of people on a consecutive and daily basis[71,72]—in which sleep is restricted to 3 to 7 hours of time in bed per night.[49,70,73,74]

At present, it remains unknown whether the same individuals vulnerable to the adverse effects of acute TSD are also vulnerable to chronic PSD.

The few reports comparing responses to both acute TSD and chronic PSD have used small sample sizes (9–13 subjects) and limited assessments,[70,75,76] and only one[75] has systematically studied the same subjects in both types of sleep loss.

The stable, trait-like interindividual differences observed in response to TSD[64–67]—with intraclass correlations (which express the proportion of variance in the data that is explained by systematic interindividual variability) ranging from 58% to 92% for neurobehavioral measures[64,67]—strongly suggest an underlying genetic component. Despite this link, however, relatively little is known about the genetic basis of differential vulnerability in healthy subjects undergoing deprivation. Furthermore, as mentioned earlier, because of reported differences in sleep homeostatic, physiologic, and behavioral responses to chronic PSD and acute TSD,[70,75,76] it is likely that specific candidate genes play different roles in the degree of vulnerability and/or resilience to the sleep homeostatic and neurobehavioral effects of acute TSD and chronic PSD. These compelling questions have produced a rapidly emerging and promising field of scientific investigation; recent studies have thus far focused on several select candidate genes, which are reviewed here.

PERIOD3 VNTR Polymorphism

Three related studies investigated the role of the VNTR polymorphism of the circadian gene PERIOD3 (PER3)—which shows similar allelic frequencies in African Americans and Caucasians[77,78] and is characterized by a 54-nucleotide coding region motif repeating in 4 or 5 units— in response to TSD using a small group of subjects specifically recruited for the homozygotic versions of this polymorphism. Compared with the 4-repeat allele (PER3[4/4]; 14 subjects), the longer, 5-repeat allele (PER3[5/5]; 10 subjects) was associated with higher sleep propensity including SWA in the sleep EEG both before and after TSD and worse cognitive performance, as assessed by a composite score of 12 tests, following TSD.[35] A subsequent report, using the same 24 subjects, clarified that the PER3[5/5] overall performance deficits were selective: they only occurred on certain executive function tests, and only at 2 to 4 hours following the melatonin rhythm peak, from approximately 6 to 8 AM.[36] Such performance differences were hypothesized to be mediated by sleep homeostasis.[35,36] Another publication using the same subjects showed that PER3[5/5] subjects had more slow-wave sleep and elevated sympathetic predominance, and a reduction of parasympathetic

activity during baseline sleep.[79] These studies found no significant differences in the melatonin and cortisol circadian rhythms, PER3 mRNA levels, or in a self-report morningness-eveningness measure,[35,36] although another study using these same subjects found PER3 expression and sleep timing were more strongly correlated in PER3[5/5] subjects.[80]

A recent neuroimaging study found that 27 healthy subjects categorized according to homozygosity for the PER3 VNTR genotype (15 PER3[4/4] subjects, 12 PER3[5/5] subjects) showed markedly different cerebral blood flow profiles using blood oxygenation level dependent functional magnetic resonance imaging (BOLD fMRI) and corresponding differences in vulnerability of executive function performance in response to TSD.[81] More studies examining the relationship of the neural mechanisms mediating trait-like differential vulnerability to sleep deprivation with selective candidate genes (beyond the PER3 VNTR polymorphism) are warranted.

The PER3 findings in TSD may not generalize to responses to chronic PSD. A recent study evaluated whether the PER3 VNTR polymorphism contributed to sleep homeostatic responses and cumulative neurobehavioral deficits during chronic PSD in PER3[4/4], PER3[4/5], and PER3[5/5] healthy adults.[49] During chronic PSD, PER3[5/5] subjects had slightly but reliably elevated sleep homeostatic pressure as measured by non-REM slow-wave energy (SWE) compared with PER3[4/4] subjects (**Fig. 1**). The PER3[4/4], PER3[4/5], and PER3[5/5] genotypes also demonstrated large, but equivalent cumulative increases in sleepiness and cumulative decreases in cognitive performance and physiologic alertness, with increasing daily intersubject variability in all genotypes. In contrast to the aforementioned data in TSD,[35,36] the PER3 VNTR variants did not differ in baseline sleep measures or in physiologic sleepiness, cognitive and executive functioning, or subjective responses to chronic PSD. Thus, the PER3 VNTR polymorphism does not appear to be a genetic marker of differential vulnerability to the cumulative neurobehavioral effects of chronic PSD. It remains possible, however, that the PER3[5/5] genotype may contribute to differential neurobehavioral vulnerability to acute TSD because it involves wakefulness at a specific circadian time in the early-morning hours (6–8 AM), when subjects in the PSD study were asleep.[49]

DQB1*0602 Allele

The human leukocyte antigen DQB1*0602 allele is closely associated with narcolepsy, a sleep

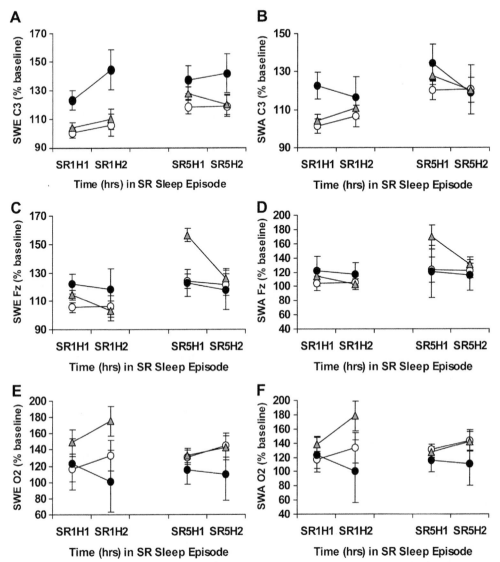

Fig. 1. Slow-wave energy (SWE) and slow-wave activity (SWA) during chronic partial sleep deprivation for the *PER3* genotypes. Mean (±SEM) hourly SWE and SWA as a percentage of baseline at the same corresponding hour derived from the C3 (*A, B*), Fz (*C, D*), or O2 (*E, F*) channels at partial sleep deprivation/restriction night 1 (SR1) and partial sleep deprivation/restriction night 5 (SR5) for hour 1 (H1) and hour 2 (H2) in *PER3*[4/4] (*open circles*), *PER3*[4/5] (*gray triangles*), and *PER3*[5/5] (*closed circles*) subjects. SWE derived from C3 (but not from Fz or O2) was significantly higher during chronic partial sleep deprivation in *PER3*[5/5] compared with *PER3*[4/4] and *PER3*[4/5] subjects. (*From* Goel N, Banks S, Mignot E, et al. PER3 polymorphism predicts cumulative sleep homeostatic but not neurobehavioral changes to chronic partial sleep deprivation. PLoS One 2009;4:e5874.)

disorder characterized by excessive daytime sleepiness, fragmented sleep, and shortened REM latency, although it is neither necessary nor sufficient for its development.[82,83]

In one large study, *DQB1*0602*-positive healthy sleepers showed shorter nighttime REM sleep latency, greater sleep continuity, and more REM sleep, but no differences in daytime sleepiness.[82] Positivity for *DQB1*0602* also was related to

more sleep-onset REM sleep periods and greater REM sleep duration during naps.[84] Thus, *DQB1*0602*-positive subjects displayed subclinical presentations of some sleep features that were reminiscent of narcolepsy.

A 2010 study evaluated whether *DQB1*0602* was a novel biomarker of differential vulnerability to homeostatic, sleepiness, and neurobehavioral deficits during chronic PSD in healthy

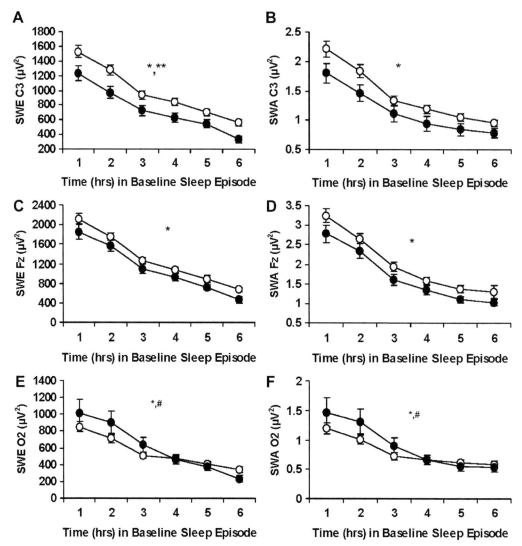

Fig. 2. Hourly slow-wave energy (SWE) and slow-wave activity (SWA) during baseline for the *DQB1*0602* groups. Mean (±SEM) hourly SWE and SWA derived from the C3 (*A, B*), Fz (*C, D*), or O2 (*E, F*) channels during baseline for *DQB1*0602*-negative subjects (*open circles*) and *DQB1*0602*-positive subjects (*closed circles*). SWE derived from C3 was lower in *DQB1*0602*-positive subjects (denoted by *double asterisk*, **$P<.05$); SWA derived from C3 and SWE and SWA derived from the Fz channel showed similar trends. As expected, SWE and SWA showed a typical pattern of dissipation across the baseline night in all 3 channels for both groups (denoted by *single asterisk*, *$P<.05$); moreover, *DQB1*0602*-positive subjects demonstrated sharper declines in sleep pressure derived from the O2 channel during the first few hours of the night than *DQB1*0602*-negative subjects (denoted by *hatch*, #$P<.05$). In some records, EEG signal quality was insufficient or contained too much artifact for reliable power spectral analysis. Thus, the final sample sizes were: for C3, *DQB1*0602* negative (n = 68) and positive (n = 24) subjects; for Fz, *DQB1*0602* negative (n = 70) and positive (n = 28) subjects; for O2, *DQB1*0602* negative (n = 74) and positive (n = 27) subjects. (*From* Goel N, Banks S, Mignot E, et al. DQB1*0602 predicts interindividual differences in physiologic sleep, sleepiness and fatigue. Neurology 2010;75:1509–19; with permission.)

sleepers positive and negative for *DQB1*0602*.[73] *DQB1*0602*-positive subjects showed decreased sleep homeostatic pressure with differentially steeper declines (**Fig. 2**), and greater sleepiness and fatigue during baseline. During chronic PSD, positive subjects displayed SWE elevation comparable to negative subjects (**Fig. 3**), despite higher sleepiness and fatigue. *DQB1*0602*-positive subjects also had more fragmented sleep during baseline and PSD, and showed differentially greater REM sleep latency reductions and smaller stage 2 reductions, along with differentially

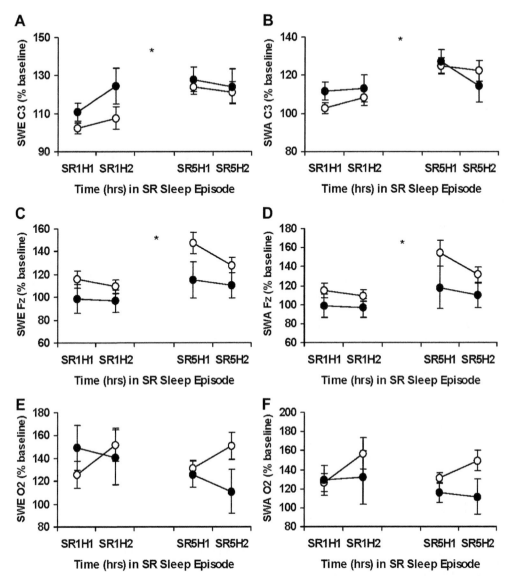

Fig. 3. Slow-wave energy (SWE) and slow-wave activity (SWA) during chronic partial sleep deprivation for the *DQB1*0602* groups. Mean (±SEM) hourly SWE and SWA as a percentage of baseline at the same corresponding hour derived from the C3 (*A, B*), Fz (*C, D*), or O2 (*E, F*) channels at partial sleep deprivation/restriction night 1 (SR1) and partial sleep deprivation/restriction night 5 (SR5) for hour 1 (H1) and hour 2 (H2) for *DQB1*0602*-negative subjects (*open circles*) and *DQB1*0602*-positive subjects (*closed circles*). SWE and SWA increased from SR1 to SR5 for the C3 and Fz channels (denoted by *single asterisk*, *$P<.05$*). There were no group differences or differential changes across nights. In some records, EEG signal quality was insufficient or contained too much artifact for reliable power spectral analysis. Thus, the final sample sizes were: for SR1 and SR5 C3, *DQB1*0602* negative ($n = 72$) and positive ($n = 28$) subjects; for SR1 and SR5 Fz, *DQB1*0602* negative ($n = 72$) and positive ($n = 27$) subjects; for SR1 and SR5 O2, *DQB1*0602* negative ($n = 72$) and positive ($n = 26$) subjects. (*From* Goel N, Banks S, Mignot E, et al. DQB1*0602 predicts interindividual differences in physiologic sleep, sleepiness and fatigue. Neurology 2010;75:1509–19; with permission.)

greater increases in fatigue. Both groups demonstrated comparable cumulative decreases in cognitive performance and increases in physiologic sleepiness to chronic PSD, and did not differ on executive function tasks.

Thus, *DQB1*0602* is associated with interindividual differences in sleep homeostasis, physiologic sleep, sleepiness, and fatigue, but not cognitive responses, during baseline and PSD. *DQB1*0602* may be a genetic marker for predicting such individual differences in both basal (fully rested) and sleep loss conditions; moreover, its positivity in healthy subjects may represent a continuum of some sleep-wake features of narcolepsy. The influence of the *DQB1*0602* allele on sleep homeostatic and neurobehavioral responses has not yet been examined in healthy subjects undergoing acute TSD, or replicated in an independent sample of individuals undergoing chronic PSD.

Catechol-O-Methyltransferase (COMT) Val158Met Polymorphism

The valine158methionine (Val158Met) polymorphism of the *catechol-O-methyltransferase* (*COMT* gene) replaces valine (*Val*) with methionine (*Met*) at codon 158 of the *COMT* protein. As a result of this common substitution, activity of the *COMT* enzyme, which modulates dopaminergic catabolism in the prefrontal cortex (PFC), is reduced 3- to 4-fold in *COMT Met* carriers compared with *Val* carriers, translating into more dopamine availability at the receptors and higher cortical dopamine concentrations.[85] This *COMT* polymorphism predicts less efficient prefrontal cortex functioning and poorer working memory performance in healthy subjects[86–89] who have the high-activity *Val* allele.

In sleep and neurodegenerative disorders, the *COMT* Val158Met polymorphism has been linked to daytime sleepiness. *Val/Val* female narcoleptic patients fell asleep 2 times faster than the *Val/Met* or *Met/Met* genotypes during the multiple sleep latency test (MSLT), while the opposite was true for males.[90] *Met/Met* narcoleptic patients also showed more sleep-onset REM periods during the MSLT, while *Val/Val* subjects showed less sleep paralysis[90] and were more responsive to modafinil's stimulating effects.[91] *Met/Met* and *Val/Met* Parkinson disease subjects demonstrated higher subjective daytime sleepiness than *Val/Val* subjects.[92]

In healthy men, the *COMT* Val158Met polymorphism is associated with sleep physiology. In acute TSD, the polymorphism predicted interindividual differences in brain alpha oscillations in wakefulness and 11- to 13-Hz EEG activity in wakefulness, REM sleep, and non-REM sleep.[93] It also modulated the effects of the wake-promoting drug modafinil on subjective well-being, sustained vigilant attention and executive functioning, and on 3.0- to 6.75-Hz and >16.75-Hz activity in non-REM sleep, but was not associated with subjective sleepiness, SWA, or slow-wave sleep changes in recovery sleep following TSD or at baseline.[94,95] Studies are underway to investigate whether the *COMT* Val158Met polymorphism contributes to

sleep homeostatic and cumulative neurobehavioral responses during basal (fully rested) conditions and during chronic PSD in *Met/Met*, *Val/Met*, and *Val/Val* healthy adult sleepers.

Adenosine-Related Polymorphisms

Other studies have investigated the role of select adenosine-related candidate genes in individual differences and in response to acute TSD. Rétey and colleagues[96] found that the 22G → A polymorphism of the adenosine deaminase gene (*ADA*) was associated with enhanced slow-wave sleep and non-REM SWA, contributing to interindividual variability in baseline sleep. Specifically, individuals with the *G/A* genotype (7 subjects) showed 30 minutes more slow-wave sleep than subjects with the *G/G* genotype (7 subjects) and, consistent with this finding, SWA was higher in *G/A* than *G/G* subjects. It is notable that this study did not test responses of these individuals to sleep deprivation, and thus it remains unknown whether these genotypes show differential sleep homeostatic responses under evoked phenotypic deprivation conditions. This group also found that the c.1083T>C polymorphism of the adenosine A2A receptor gene (*ADORA2A*) is related to objective and subjective differences in the effects of caffeine on non-REM sleep after TSD[97] and is associated with individual differences in various measures of baseline EEG during sleep and wakefulness.[96] While promising, replication of these data in independent samples is needed; in addition, the role of these two genetic variants in response to chronic PSD has not yet been established.

Thus, several common genetic polymorphisms involved in circadian, sleep-wake, and cognitive regulation appear to underlie interindividual differences in basal (fully rested) sleep parameters and homeostatic regulation of sleep in response to sleep deprivation (both chronic PSD and acute TSD) in healthy adults.

GENOME-WIDE ASSOCIATION STUDIES OF HUMAN SLEEP

To date, only one study has employed a genome-wide association approach to examine phenotypic-genotypic interactions in healthy human sleepers.[98] Moderate heritability estimates for self-rated sleepiness (29%; assessed by the Epworth Sleepiness Scale) and for habitual sleep duration (17%) and habitual bedtime (22%), assessed by a standard questionnaire used in the Sleep Heart Health Study, were found in 749 subjects. The genome-wide analysis revealed that habitual bedtime and sleep duration were modulated by genetic loci containing circadian clock-related genes including casein kinase 2A2 (CSNK2A2), prokineticin 2 (PROK2), and CLOCK. Furthermore, genes encoding NPSRI and PDE4D were identified as possible mediators of habitual bedtime and subjective sleepiness, respectively. While intriguing, these data need to be replicated and extended to studies that include physiologic measures of sleep.

FUTURE DIRECTIONS

With the exception of two recent studies,[49,73] all candidate gene studies involving sleep physiologic and neurobehavioral responses to sleep loss have used small sample sizes (14–24 subjects) and have only examined homozygotic individuals.[35,36,93,94,96,97] Larger sample sizes and assessment of phenotype-genotype relationships in both homozygous and heterozygous individuals are needed to definitively determine whether such candidate genes involved in regulation of sleep-wake, circadian, and cognitive functions are associated with interindividual neurobehavioral responses to sleep loss across an entire population. This approach is particularly critical because individuals are necessarily categorized into different genotypes, reducing sample sizes in each subgroup. Future candidate gene studies therefore must consistently use sample sizes in the hundreds, rather than tens, to detect statistically reliable differences across genotypes.

In addition, replication of findings in independent samples is needed to determine whether findings are genuine and are not due to chance; ideally, studies should also be replicated in different ethnic groups to increase generalizability of the findings. Genome-wide association studies using physiologic sleep measures as outcomes are also needed to assess basal (fully rested) individual differences as well as responses to sleep deprivation; however, these will likely require obtaining data in several laboratories, given the expense, time, and effort needed to conduct such rigorous studies.

Searching for genetic markers of basal sleep measures and of sleep homeostatic and neurobehavioral differential vulnerability to sleep deprivation is an active and profitable area of research. Among other advantages, identification of such markers will provide a viable means to determine those individuals in the general population who may need more habitual sleep or who may need to prevent or mitigate sleep deprivation through lifestyle choices and effective interventions and countermeasures.

REFERENCES

1. Van Dongen HP, Dinges DF. Investigating the interaction between the homeostatic and circadian processes of sleep-wake regulation for the prediction of waking neurobehavioral performance. J Sleep Res 2003;12:181–7.
2. Goel N, Van Dongen HP, Dinges DF. Circadian rhythms in sleepiness, alertness, and performance. In: Kryger MH, Dement WC, Roth T, editors. Principles and practice of sleep medicine. 5th edition. Philadelphia: Elsevier; 2011. p. 445–55.
3. Achermann P, Dijk DJ, Brunner DP, et al. A model of human sleep homeostasis based on EEG slow-wave activity; quantitative comparison of data and simulations. Brain Res Bull 1993;31:97–113.
4. Borbély AA. A two process model of sleep regulation. Hum Neurobiol 1982;1:195–204.
5. Mallis MM, Mejdal S, Nguyen TT, et al. Summary of the key features of seven biomathematical models of human fatigue and performance. Aviat Space Environ Med 2004;75:A4–14.
6. Daan S, Beersma DGM, Borbély AA. Timing of human sleep: recovery process gated by a circadian pacemaker. Am J Physiol 1984;246:R161–78.
7. Achermann P, Borbély AA. Simulation of daytime vigilance by the additive interaction of a homeostatic and a circadian process. Biol Cybern 1994;71:115–21.
8. Khalsa SBS, Jewett ME, Duffy JF, et al. The timing of the human circadian clock is accurately represented by the core body temperature rhythm following phase shifts to a three-cycle light stimulus near the critical zone. J Biol Rhythms 2000;15:524–30.
9. Edgar DM, Dement WC, Fuller CA. Effect of SCN lesions on sleep in squirrel monkeys: evidence for opponent processes in sleep-wake regulation. J Neurosci 1993;13:1065–79.
10. Doran SM, Van Dongen HPA, Dinges DF. Sustained attention performance during sleep deprivation: evidence of state instability. Arch Ital Biol 2001;139:253–67.
11. Kerkhof GA, Van Dongen HPA. Morning-type and evening-type individuals differ in the phase position of their endogenous circadian oscillator. Neurosci Lett 1996;218:153–6.
12. Baehr EK, Revelle W, Eastman CI. Individual differences in the phase and amplitude of the human circadian temperature rhythm: with an emphasis on morningness-eveningness. J Sleep Res 2000;9:117–27.
13. Horne JA, Östberg O. A self-assessment questionnaire to determine morningness–eveningness in human circadian rhythms. Int J Chronobiol 1976;4:97–110.
14. Smith CS, Reilly D, Midkiff K. Evaluation of three circadian rhythm questionnaires with suggestions

for an improved measure of morningness. J Appl Psychol 1989;74:728–38.

15. Roenneberg T, Wirz-Justice A, Merrow M. Life between clocks: daily temporal patterns of human chronotypes. J Biol Rhythms 2003;18:80–90.

16. Roenneberg T, Kuehnle T, Juda M, et al. Epidemiology of the human circadian clock. Sleep Med Rev 2007;11:429–38.

17. Duffy JF, Dijk D-J, Klerman EB, et al. Later endogenous circadian temperature nadir relative to an earlier wake time in older people. Am J Physiol 1998;275:R1478–87.

18. Foster RG, Roenneberg T. Human responses to the geophysical daily, annual and lunar cycles. Curr Biol 2008;18:R784–94.

19. Adan A, Natale V. Gender differences in morningness-eveningness preference. Chronobiol Int 2002;19:709–20.

20. Randler C. Gender differences in morningness-eveningness assessed by self-report questionnaires: a meta-analysis. Pers Indiv Differ 2007;43:1667–75.

21. Hur Y-M. Stability of genetic influence on morningness-eveningness: a cross-sectional examination of South Korean twins from preadolescence to young adulthood. J Sleep Res 2007;16:17–23.

22. Hur YM, Bouchard TJ Jr, Lykken DT. Genetic and environmental influence on morningness-eveningness. Pers Indiv Differ 1998;25:917–25.

23. Vink JM, Groot AS, Kerkhof GA, et al. Genetic analysis of morningness and eveningness. Chronobiol Int 2001;18:809–22.

24. Van Dongen HP, Kerkhof GA, Dinges DF. Human circadian rhythms. In: Sehgal A, editor. Molecular biology of circadian rhythms. New York: John Wiley and Sons; 2004. p. 255–69.

25. Takahashi JS, Hong HK, Ko CH, et al. The genetics of mammalian circadian order and disorder: implications for physiology and disease. Nat Rev Genet 2008;9:764–75.

26. Katzenberg D, Young T, Finn L, et al. A CLOCK polymorphism associated with human diurnal preference. Sleep 1998;21:569–76.

27. Mishima K, Tozawa T, Satoh K, et al. The 3111T/C polymorphism of hClock is associated with evening preference and delayed sleep timing in a Japanese population sample. Am J Med Genet B Neuropsychiatr Genet 2005;133:101–4.

28. Robilliard DL, Archer SN, Arendt J, et al. The 3111 Clock gene polymorphism is not associated with sleep and circadian rhythmicity in phenotypically characterized human subjects. J Sleep Res 2002;11:305–12.

29. Iwase T, Kajimura N, Uchiyama M, et al. Mutation screening of the human Clock gene in circadian rhythm sleep disorders. Psychiatry Res 2002;109:121–8.

30. Pedrazzoli M, Louzada FM, Pereira DS, et al. Clock polymorphisms and circadian rhythms phenotypes in a sample of the Brazilian population. Chronobiol Int 2007;24:1–8.

31. Archer SN, Robilliard DL, Skene DJ, et al. A length polymorphism in the circadian clock gene PER3 is linked to delayed sleep phase syndrome and extreme diurnal preference. Sleep 2003;26:413–5.

32. Pereira DS, Tufik S, Louzada FM, et al. Association of the length polymorphism in the human PER3 gene with the delayed sleep-phase syndrome: does latitude have an influence upon it? Sleep 2005;28:29–32.

33. Jones KH, Ellis J, von Schantz M, et al. Age-related change in the association between a polymorphism in the PER3 gene and preferred timing of sleep and waking activities. J Sleep Res 2007;16:12–6.

34. Ebisawa T, Uchiyama M, Kajimura N, et al. Association of structural polymorphisms in the human period3 gene with delayed sleep phase syndrome. EMBO Rep 2001;2:342–6.

35. Viola AU, Archer SN, James LM, et al. PER3 polymorphism predicts sleep structure and waking performance. Curr Biol 2007;17:613–8.

36. Groeger JA, Viola AU, Lo JC, et al. Early morning executive functioning during sleep deprivation is compromised by a PERIOD3 polymorphism. Sleep 2008;31:1159–67.

37. Carpen JD, Archer SN, Skene DJ, et al. A single-nucleotide polymorphism in the 5'-untranslated region of the hPER2 gene is associated with diurnal preference. J Sleep Res 2005;14:293–7.

38. Carpen JD, von Schantz M, Smits M, et al. A silent polymorphism in the PER1 gene associates with extreme diurnal preference in humans. J Hum Genet 2006;51:1122–5.

39. American Academy of Sleep Medicine. The international classification of sleep disorders: diagnostic and coding manual. 2nd edition. Westchester (IL): American Academy of Sleep Medicine; 2005.

40. Sack RL, Auckley D, Auger RR, et al. Circadian rhythm sleep disorders: part II, advanced sleep phase disorder, delayed sleep phase disorder, free-running disorder, and irregular sleep-wake rhythm. An American Academy of Sleep Medicine review. Sleep 2007;30:1484–501.

41. Campbell SS, Murphy PJ. Delayed sleep phase disorder in temporal isolation. Sleep 2007;30:1225–8.

42. Takano A, Uchiyama M, Kajimura N, et al. A missense variation in human casein kinase I epsilon gene that induces functional alteration and shows an inverse association with circadian rhythm sleep disorders. Neuropsychopharmacology 2004;29:1901–9.

43. Reid KJ, Chang AM, Dubocovich ML, et al. Familial advanced sleep phase syndrome. Arch Neurol 2001;58:1089–94.

44. Jones CR, Campbell SS, Zone SE, et al. Familial advanced sleep-phase syndrome: a short-period circadian rhythm variant in humans. Nat Med 1999; 5:1062–5.

45. Toh KL, Jones CR, He Y, et al. An hPer2 phosphorylation site mutation in familial advanced sleep phase syndrome. Science 2001;291:1040–3.

46. Satoh K, Mishima K, Inoue Y, et al. Two pedigrees of familial advanced sleep phase syndrome in Japan. Sleep 2003;26:416–7.

47. Xu Y, Padiath QS, Shapiro RE, et al. Functional consequences of a CKIdelta mutation causing familial advanced sleep phase syndrome. Nature 2005;434:640–4.

48. Kerkhof GA. Inter-individual differences in the human circadian system: a review. Biol Psychol 1985;20:83–112.

49. Goel N, Banks S, Mignot E, et al. PER3 polymorphism predicts cumulative sleep homeostatic but not neurobehavioral changes to chronic partial sleep deprivation. PLoS ONE 2009;4:e5874.

50. Dauvilliers Y, Maret S, Tafti M. Genetics of normal and pathological sleep in humans. Sleep Med Rev 2005;9:91–100.

51. Tafti M, Maret S, Dauvilliers Y. Genes for normal sleep and sleep disorders. Ann Med 2005;37:580–9.

52. Tafti M. Genetic aspects of normal and disturbed sleep. Sleep Med 2009;10(Suppl 1):S17–21.

53. Ambrosius U, Lietzenmaier S, Wehrle R, et al. Heritability of sleep electroencephalogram. Biol Psychiatry 2008;64:344–8.

54. De Gennaro L, Marzano C, Fratello F, et al. The electroencephalographic fingerprint of sleep is genetically determined: a twin study. Ann Neurol 2008; 64:455–60.

55. Werth E, Achermann P, Dijk DJ, et al. Spindle frequency activity in the sleep EEG: individual differences and topographic distribution. Electroencephalogr Clin Neurophysiol 1997;103:535–42.

56. Tan X, Campbell IG, Palagini L, et al. High internight reliability of computer-measured NREM delta, sigma, and beta: biological implications. Biol Psychiatry 2000;48:1010–9.

57. Finelli LA, Achermann P, Borbely AA. Individual 'fingerprints' in human sleep EEG topography. Neuropsychopharmacology 2001;25:S57–62.

58. De Gennaro L, Ferrara M, Vecchio F, et al. An electroencephalographic fingerprint of human sleep. Neuroimage 2005;26:114–22.

59. Tucker AM, Dinges DF, Van Dongen HP. Trait interindividual differences in the sleep physiology of healthy young adults. J Sleep Res 2007;16:170–80.

60. Buckelmuller J, Landolt HP, Stassen HH, et al. Trait-like individual differences in the human sleep electroencephalogram. Neuroscience 2006;138:351–6.

61. Andretic R, Franken P, Tafti M. Genetics of sleep. Annu Rev Genet 2008;42:361–88.

62. He Y, Jones CR, Fujiki N, et al. The transcriptional repressor DEC2 regulates sleep length in mammals. Science 2009;325:866–70.

63. Guindalini C, Martins RC, Andersen ML, et al. Influence of genotype on dopamine transporter availability in human striatum and sleep architecture. Psychiatry Res 2010;179:238–40.

64. Van Dongen HP, Baynard MD, Maislin G, et al. Systematic interindividual differences in neurobehavioral impairment from sleep loss: evidence of trait-like differential vulnerability. Sleep 2004;27:423–33.

65. Leproult R, Colecchia EF, Berardi AM, et al. Individual differences in subjective and objective alertness during sleep deprivation are stable and unrelated. Am J Physiol Regul Integr Comp Physiol 2003;284:R280–90.

66. Van Dongen HP, Dinges DF. Sleep, circadian rhythms, and psychomotor vigilance performance. Clin Sports Med 2005;24:237–49.

67. Van Dongen HP, Maislin G, Dinges DF. Dealing with interindividual differences in the temporal dynamics of fatigue and performance: importance and techniques. Aviat Space Environ Med 2004; 75(3 Suppl):A147–54.

68. Frey DJ, Badia P, Wright KP Jr. Inter- and intra-individual variability in performance near the circadian nadir during sleep deprivation. J Sleep Res 2004;13:305–15.

69. Van Dongen HP, Dijkman MV, Maislin G, et al. Phenotypic aspect of vigilance decrement during sleep deprivation. Physiologist 1999;42:A-5.

70. Van Dongen HP, Maislin G, Mullington JM, et al. The cumulative cost of additional wakefulness: dose-response effects on neurobehavioral functions and sleep physiology from chronic sleep restriction and total sleep deprivation. Sleep 2003;26:117–26.

71. Banks S, Dinges DF. Behavioral and physiological consequences of sleep restriction in humans. J Clin Sleep Med 2007;3:519–28.

72. Goel N, Rao H, Durmer JS, et al. Neurocognitive consequences of sleep deprivation. Semin Neurol 2009;29:320–39.

73. Goel N, Banks S, Mignot E, et al. DQB1*0602 predicts interindividual differences in physiologic sleep, sleepiness and fatigue. Neurology 2010;75: 1509–19.

74. Bliese PD, Wesensten NJ, Balkin TJ. Age and individual variability in performance during sleep restriction. J Sleep Res 2006;15:376–85.

75. Drake CL, Roehrs TA, Burduvali E, et al. Effects of rapid versus slow accumulation of eight hours of sleep loss. Psychophysiology 2001;38:979–87.

76. Rowland LM, Thomas ML, Thorne DR, et al. Oculomotor responses during partial and total sleep deprivation. Aviat Space Environ Med 2005;76:C104–13.

77. Nadkarni NA, Weale ME, von Schantz M, et al. Evolution of a length polymorphism in the human

PER3 gene, a component of the circadian system. J Biol Rhythms 2005;20:490–9.

78. Ciarleglio CM, Ryckman KK, Servick SV, et al. Genetic differences in human circadian clock genes among worldwide populations. J Biol Rhythms 2008; 23:330–40.

79. Viola AU, James LM, Archer SN, et al. PER3 polymorphism and cardiac autonomic control: effects of sleep debt and circadian phase. Am J Physiol Heart Circ Physiol 2008;295:H2156–63.

80. Archer SN, Viola AU, Kyriakopoulou V, et al. Interindividual differences in habitual sleep timing and entrained phase of endogenous circadian rhythms of BMAL1, PER2 and PER3 mRNA in human leukocytes. Sleep 2008;31:608–17.

81. Vandewalle G, Archer SN, Wuillaume C, et al. Functional magnetic resonance imaging-assessed brain responses during an executive task depend on interaction of sleep homeostasis, circadian phase, and PER3 genotype. J Neurosci 2009;29:7948–56.

82. Mignot E, Young T, Lin L, et al. Nocturnal sleep and daytime sleepiness in normal subjects with HLA-DQB1*0602. Sleep 1999;22:347–52.

83. Dauvilliers Y, Tafti M. Molecular genetics and treatment of narcolepsy. Ann Med 2006;38:252–62.

84. Mignot E, Lin L, Finn L, et al. Correlates of sleep-onset REM periods during the Multiple Sleep Latency Test in community adults. Brain 2006;129:1609–23.

85. Tunbridge EM, Harrison PJ, Weinberger DR. Catechol-o-methyltransferase, cognition, and psychosis: Val158-Met and beyond. Biol Psychiatry 2006;60:141–51.

86. Savitz J, Solms M, Ramesar R. The molecular genetics of cognition: dopamine, COMT and BDNF. Genes Brain Behav 2006;5:311–28.

87. Egan MF, Goldberg TE, Kolachana BS, et al. Effect of COMT Val108/158 Met genotype on frontal lobe function and risk for schizophrenia. Proc Natl Acad Sci U S A 2001;98:6917–22.

88. Dickinson D, Elvevåg B. Genes, cognition and brain through a COMT lens. Neuroscience 2009;164:72–87.

89. Barnett JH, Jones PB, Robbins TW, et al. Effects of the catechol-O-methyltransferase Val158Met polymorphism on executive function: a meta-analysis of the Wisconsin Card Sort Test in schizophrenia and healthy controls. Mol Psychiatry 2007;12:502–9.

90. Dauvilliers Y, Neidhart E, Lecendreux M, et al. MAO-A and COMT polymorphisms and gene effects in narcolepsy. Mol Psychiatry 2001;6:367–72.

91. Dauvilliers Y, Neidhart E, Billiard M, et al. Sexual dimorphism of the catechol-O-methyltransferase gene in narcolepsy is associated with response to modafinil. Pharmacogenomics J 2002;2:65–8.

92. Frauscher B, Högl B, Maret S, et al. Association of daytime sleepiness with COMT polymorphism in patients with Parkinson disease: a pilot study. Sleep 2004;27:733–6.

93. Bodenmann S, Rusterholz T, Dürr R, et al. The functional Val158Met polymorphism of COMT predicts interindividual differences in brain α oscillations in young men. J Neurosci 2009;29:10855–62.

94. Bodenmann S, Xu S, Luhmann U, et al. Pharmacogenetics of modafinil after sleep loss: Catechol-O-methyltransferase genotype modulates waking functions but not recovery sleep. Clin Pharmacol Ther 2009;85:296–304.

95. Bodenmann S, Landolt HP. Effects of modafinil on the sleep EEG depend on Val158Met genotype of COMT. Sleep 2010;33:1027–35.

96. Rétey JV, Adam M, Honegger E, et al. A functional genetic variation of adenosine deaminase affects the duration and intensity of deep sleep in humans. Proc Natl Acad Sci U S A 2005;102:15676–81.

97. Rétey JV, Adam M, Khatami R, et al. A genetic variation in the adenosine A2A receptor gene (ADOR-A2A) contributes to individual sensitivity to caffeine effects on sleep. Clin Pharmacol Ther 2007;81: 692–8.

98. Gottlieb DJ, O'Connor GT, Wilk JB. Genome-wide association of sleep and circadian phenotypes. BMC Med Genet 2007;8(Suppl 1):S9.

Genetics of Circadian Rhythm Disorders

Anne-Marie Chang, PhD[a,b],*, Phyllis Zee, MD, PhD[c]

KEYWORDS
- Advanced sleep phase • Circadian rhythm sleep disorders
- Delayed sleep phase • Genetics • Human circadian rhythms

CIRCADIAN RHYTHMS IN MAMMALS

The circadian timing system is ubiquitous to nearly all organisms on earth. The 24-hour cycle of light/dark exhibited by the solar day is reflected in a myriad of circadian rhythms in many living organisms. External environmental changes in the 24-hour day synchronize the various physiologic, biochemical, and behavioral processes in a predictable pattern. The mammalian circadian pacemaker, or biological clock, is located in the suprachiasmatic nucleus (SCN) of the anterior hypothalamus. This circadian clock synchronizes internal biological processes to external time cues and maintains the temporal organization of these processes with each other. This type of circadian organization with respect to the external environment establishes temporal categories in which animals are active or at rest, and may have evolved in response to different needs of organisms (eg, availability of food) and reduced competition for resources. One such circadian rhythm is the timing of the sleep/wake cycle. The daily patterns of light and dark signals entrain the circadian clock as to the appropriate time for sleep.

As a diurnal species, human beings generally prefer to schedule activities during the daytime and sleep at night. Diurnal preference, the proclivity to schedule activity for certain times of the day, varies in the general population. Individuals who prefer to be active in the early part of the day (morning types) are often called larks and those who have a preference for nighttime activity (evening types) are known as owls. Many individuals, if not most, have a neither type diurnal preference. In the past 40 years several questionnaires have been developed and used to subjectively assess diurnal preference. Although they may have been originally developed to identify workers' tolerance of and abilities to adjust to changing work schedules, these questionnaires have become valuable research tools in examining the differences underlying morningness or eveningness and various influences on sleep timing. Morning and evening types have been shown to exhibit differences in circadian phase and phase angle of entrainment of body temperature and hormonal rhythms; in habitual timing of sleep and sleep propensity; and in performance measures. Diurnal preference is influenced by several environmental factors, such as work, school, and social schedules, but has also been shown to have a genetic component.

Numerous animal studies have shown that like diurnal preference, other expressions of circadian behavior have a genetic basis. The investigation of circadian mutants and homologs of circadian genes, originally identified in nonmammalian organisms, led to identification of the genetic components of the mammalian circadian pacemaker. This molecular mechanism consists of autoregulatory feedback loops of genes that regulate circadian timing at the levels of transcription, translation, and posttranslation; and shows remarkable conservation in many species,

[a] Division of Sleep Medicine, Harvard Medical School, 221 Longwood Avenue, Boston, MA 02115, USA
[b] Department of Medicine, Brigham and Women's Hospital, 221 Longwood Avenue, Boston, MA 02115, USA
[c] Department of Neurology, Northwestern University Feinberg School of Medicine, 710 North Lake Shore Drive, Chicago, IL 60611, USA
* Corresponding author. Division of Sleep Medicine, Harvard Medical School, 221 Longwood Avenue, Boston, MA 02115.
E-mail address: amchang@rics.bwh.harvard.edu

Sleep Med Clin 6 (2011) 183–190
doi:10.1016/j.jsmc.2011.03.002
1556-407X/11/$ – see front matter © 2011 Elsevier Inc. All rights reserved.

including humans (**Fig. 1**). The genes that make up this mammalian molecular clock are essential to the generation of circadian rhythms, and mutations in these genes have been shown to result in loss of or alterations in these daily rhythms. Genetic components of this clock mechanism are found ubiquitously throughout various tissues suggesting that peripheral clocks play key roles in the maintenance of circadian alignment. Therefore, alterations of the molecular machinery are likely to affect multiple organ systems, in addition to the brain, which has implications for health that go beyond sleep and performance.

CIRCADIAN RHYTHM SLEEP DISORDERS

Sleep is essential for health and performance. As a physiologic and behavioral process, sleep is markedly conserved in numerous species and seems to fulfill multiple functions. Sleep loss, whether the result of insufficiency, disruption, or impairment, has serious implications for general health, mood, behavior, and cognitive performance. Acute and chronic sleep deprivation results in impairment of cardiometabolic function, cognitive performance, and mood.

The timing of sleep is critical to the duration and quality of sleep. For optimal sleep, the major sleep episode should be aligned with the circadian timing of sleep propensity. When the sleep homeostatic process and the circadian pacemaker are misaligned, sleep is disrupted. Habitual misalignment may result in circadian rhythm sleep disorders shown in **Fig. 2**. There are 2 categories of circadian rhythm disorders: those in which the external environment is altered relative to the internal circadian clock, such as jet lag and shift work sleep disorder; and those in which the internal clock is altered relative to the external environment, such as advanced sleep phase (ASP), delayed sleep phase (DSP), irregular sleep/wake, and nonentrained type.

Those in the first category may be temporary, as in the case of jet lag after travel across multiple time zones, which is alleviated once the circadian clock becomes reset to the external time (day/night cycle); or these conditions may be chronic, such as working a rotating shift for months or years, preventing the entrainment of sleep to a stable schedule. It is believed, however, that good sleep can be restored in individuals suffering from jet lag or shift work sleep disorder, once the external source of the misalignment is removed (eg, a shift worker quits their job or begins working a regular stable schedule). Although these disorders are environmentally or behaviorally induced, differences in the genetic regulation of circadian

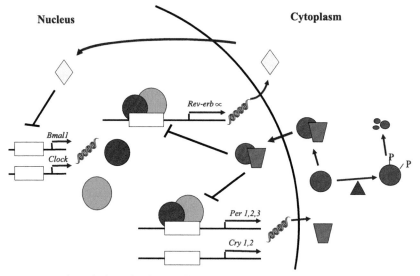

Fig. 1. The putative circadian clock molecular mechanism in mammals. Proteins of several circadian genes are color coded: CLOCK is green, BMAL1 is blue, PER are red, CRYs are orange, CKIε is purple, and REV-ERBα is yellow. CLOCK and BMAL1 are transcription factors that dimerize to initiate transcription of *Period* and *Cryptochrome* genes. PER and CRY proteins dimerize in the cytoplasm, reenter the nucleus, and negatively disrupt the CLOCK-BMAL1 complex to ultimately downregulate their own transcription. Once the transcription, translation, posttranslation, dimerization, and translocation turnover occur, the cycle begins again. The time course is approximately 24 hours. Other feedback loops, positive and negative, interconnect with and regulate this central loop.

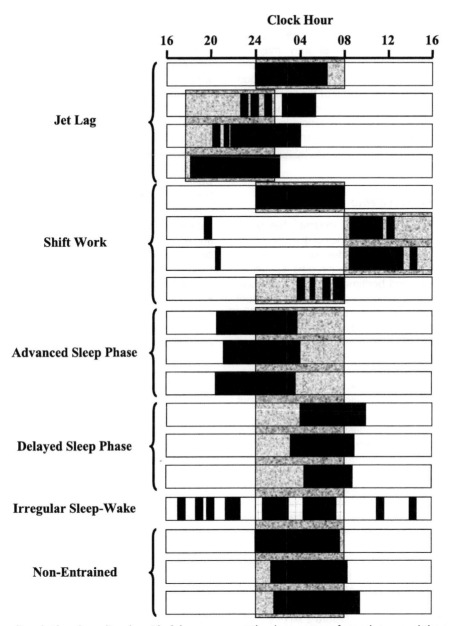

Fig. 2. Circadian rhythm sleep disorders. Black bars represent the sleep pattern for each type and the gray boxes represent possible sleep opportunities or typical sleep times. Examples are shown for jet lag, where the typical sleep time is advanced by 7 hours (trans-Atlantic flight), and for shift work, where a day shift (sleep at night) is followed by 2 consecutive night shifts (sleep during the day) followed again by a day shift (rotating shift schedule). The intrinsic circadian rhythm disorders, that is, ASP syndrome, DSP syndrome, irregular sleep-wake, and nonentrained sleep conditions, are also shown.

rhythms likely play a role in the vulnerability to jet lag and shift work disorder.

The conditions in the second category are believed to be based on chronic alterations in the circadian clock that result in a nonconventional phase relationship with the external temporal light cues. Although these conditions are related to the circadian timing of sleep, there is still little known

about how the pacemaker is altered or causes downstream changes in the regulation of sleep. DSP and ASP are the most common of the 4 types in this group, and increasing numbers of individuals are being diagnosed and studied to understand more about the pathophysiology and underlying mechanism involved, with the ultimate goal of developing effective treatments. Little is known about irregular sleep/wake or nonentrained sleep conditions as they are rare disorders. It has been suggested, however, that they may be more extreme forms of DSP, at least in the case of nonentrained sleep, and therefore elucidation of the underlying cause for any of these circadian rhythm sleep disorders may advance the treatment of others. Our goal in this article is provide a review of DSP and ASP, with particular focus on the genetic basis of these circadian rhythm sleep phase disorders.

Diagnosis and Prevalence

Based on clinical diagnostic criteria,[1] the diagnosis of either DSP or ASP includes a complaint of inability to sleep at the desired time. In the case of DSP, patients often struggle to initiate sleep at the desired bedtime and then may have restricted sleep duration because work or school demands require an early wake time. On the other hand, patients with ASP may or may not follow an early bedtime schedule, but usually complain of the inability to remain asleep until the desired wake time. The diagnostic criteria for both circadian rhythm sleep disorders requires a stable sleep pattern that is advanced or delayed but normal in quality and duration when patients are allowed to choose their desired sleep times. The advanced or delayed sleep schedule must be verified by actigraphic measurement or by sleep diary for a minimum of 1 week. Criteria for diagnosis of DSP or ASP exclude any other sleep disorder or problem, any medical or psychiatric disorder, or any use of medication or substance that can account for the habitually advanced or delayed sleep schedule.

DSP, the more common of the circadian rhythm phase disorders, was the first to be described[2] and is characterized by a sleep schedule that is consistently later than desired. Patients with DSP have difficulty falling asleep before 2 AM or waking before 10 AM. For these individuals, the preferred time of day for maximum productivity is late afternoon or evening, as is reflected on questionnaires of diurnal preference when they typically score as evening types. Although there may be reports of chronic sleep onset insomnia, the most common complaint in cases of DSP is the inability to wake sufficiently early for work or school schedules. When individuals with DSP strictly adhere to these early morning schedules, they frequently develop problems as a result of chronic sleep restriction because of the inability to sleep at a desired earlier bedtime. The usual symptom that arises from this habitual sleep schedule is excessive daytime sleepiness, particularly during the early portion of the day. This complaint may be even more common in patients with DSP because they may need more than the typical 7 to 8 hours of sleep per night.[3] To deal with this sleep deprivation, individuals with DSP often extend sleep on days off or weekends when their schedules permit. Although the prevalence of DSP is low (<1%) in the general population in several different countries,[4–6] there seems to be a higher number of cases reported among adolescents and young adults.[7,8] Evidence from several studies showing a delay in the sleep/wake rhythm in this population supports this finding.[9–11]

ASP, on the other hand, is characterized by habitual sleep and wake times that are involuntary and earlier than desired. A common complaint from patients with ASP is of early awakening or sleep maintenance insomnia; in most cases these individuals have difficulty sleeping later than 5 AM. Patients with ASP report feeling most alert in the morning and generally rate themselves as morning types on questionnaires of diurnal preference. Another complaint is sleepiness in the evening hours, particularly if familial or social demands prevent the ability to go to bed early; as a result, patients with ASP may also be chronically sleep deprived. The prevalence of ASP is estimated to be significantly lower than DSP, which is likely due to the under reporting of ASP cases. An early sleep/wake schedule may be advantageous in fitting to societal norms and schedules, and therefore people with ASP may not complain about their sleep habits or seek treatment. Furthermore, because early bedtimes and wake times are commonly seen with aging, complaints associated with ASP may be attributed to normal senescence by patients and by their health care providers. Although there may typically be an advance of the sleep schedule associated with aging, sleep also tends to be more fragmented and there is evidence of alterations in the sleep homeostat in older adults.[12] Therefore, it is unclear whether the underlying pathophysiology of age-associated advance in the timing of sleep and wake is the same as ASP in younger individuals.

Pathophysiology

Studies of patients with DSP and ASP show that, for the most part, sleep architecture and duration are essentially normal but the circadian timing of the consolidated sleep episode is altered. Based on the fundamental properties of the circadian timing system with regard to the temporal regulation of sleep, several possible underlying mechanisms could explain this persistent misalignment or altered phase relationship between the sleep/wake cycle and the external environment. Under entrained conditions, the circadian pacemaker maintains a stable phase relationship with the 24-hour time cues of the environment, namely the light/dark cycle. Given that the endogenous circadian period of humans is close to, but not exactly, 24 hours; the biological clock must make minor daily adjustments to maintain this phase angle. Light exposure occurring during the early portion of the day causes the circadian clock to reset to an earlier clock time (phase advances) and light exposure during the evening or early portion of the night induces resetting to a later time (phase delays). If, for any reason, the necessary phase shifts are not obtained, the timing of the sleep/wake cycle occurs at an altered time relative to the clock hour. One potential explanation for the altered phase angle of sleep in patients with DSP and ASP is a long or short endogenous circadian period, respectively. In the case of DSP, a long period would require daily phase advances to remain entrained to the solar day. If the circadian period were sufficiently longer than 24 hours as to require significant phase advances (ie, greater than a few minutes), this could result in an altered phase relationship and delayed sleep timing. If the endogenous period were long enough to be outside the range of entrainment to the 24 day this could cause the nonentrained sleep disorder. Likewise, with respect to ASP, a short circadian period would necessitate a daily phase delay to maintain entrainment to the external light/dark cycle; and if substantially shorter than 24 hours, could cause a subsequent advance in the sleep schedule. The report of an individual from a familial case of ASP who exhibited a short circadian period[13] supports this explanation that the endogenous period of the circadian pacemaker plays a role in the development of these circadian rhythm sleep patterns.

It is also possible that the extreme sleep schedule in cases of DSP or ASP masks the respective phase delay or phase advance regions of the phase response curve (PRC). Patients with DSP who typically stay awake during late night hours are likely being exposed to light in the delaying region of the PRC. Furthermore, by sleeping in late they are likely avoiding the morning light needed to advance the circadian timing system. A longer interval between the body temperature minimum and wake time has been reported in patients with DSP,[14] providing evidence that the sleep episode lasting later into the morning and farther from the temperature nadir would mask the advance portion of the PRC. The same could be said for individuals with ASP who consistently expose the phase advancing region of the PRC to light by the early morning sleep schedule but are less likely to receive evening light necessary for phase delays. This habitual sleep schedule leads to a perpetuating cycle of behavior of delayed or advanced sleep in individuals with DSP and ASP.

An alternative but related explanation for the delayed or advanced sleep phase in these disorders lies in the sensitivity to the entraining effects of light, described as a weak or low-amplitude portion of the PRC. Such a decrease in the sensitivity to light affects the ability to synchronize the sleep/wake rhythm to the environmental light cues. In the case of DSP, there may be a significantly small advance portion of the light PRC accounting for the reduced ability to phase advance the sleep episode to a more desired time. Increased sensitivity to light exposure during the evening/night has been shown in patients with DSP.[15] These findings indicate that an altered response to light may play an important role in these circadian rhythm phase conditions. Therefore, it is likely that not only changes in the endogenous circadian period but also light entrainment mechanisms of the circadian system contribute to the altered timing of sleep in DSP and ASP.

Contrary to the commonly believed explanation that both DSP and ASP are caused only by changes in the circadian timing of sleep; there is evidence that the sleep homeostat itself is altered in circadian rhythm sleep disorders. Some studies of polysomnographic recordings in patients with DSP who were sleeping at their desired bedtime and wake time showed normal sleep architecture relative to controls,[16,17] whereas others have found sleep disturbances in the patients compared with controls.[18] When studied on an imposed sleep schedule, patients with DSP demonstrated significantly longer sleep onset latency.[19] After 24 hours of sleep deprivation, individuals with DSP showed poor compensation for sleep loss during both the subjective day and early subjective night.[20] Furthermore, there was a larger phase angle between the phase of the melatonin onset and sleep propensity, suggesting that these two are linked in patients with DSP making it difficult for them to reset their sleep phase. Similar results were seen in a study of morning and evening types; those with intermediate circadian phases showed significant differences in the dissipation of sleep pressure compared with those with extreme circadian phases.[21] These findings implicate both the circadian timing system and the sleep homeostatic process as contributors to the regulation of sleep timing and to diurnal preference.

GENETIC BASIS OF HUMAN CIRCADIAN RHYTHM SLEEP DISORDERS

In the past several decades, research studies in animals have examined the genetic regulation of both the circadian and sleep homeostatic mechanisms. Identification of genes involved in these systems reveal complicated interactions that regulate sleep and wakefulness and contribute to the control of sleep duration and timing. The *Clock* gene was the first circadian gene identified in mammals and led to the elucidation of the autoregulatory feedback loops that make up the circadian pacemaker.[22,23] Sleep studies of *Clock* mutant mice demonstrated a decrease in sleep duration and a reduction in sleep need.[24] Similarly, studies of other circadian gene mutants, *Cry1* and *Cry2* double-knockout mice, have shown an increase in homeostatic sleep drive.[25] On the other hand, published reports investigating the sleep of m*Per1* and m*Per2* mutants revealed no difference in homeostatic sleep regulation compared with wildtype mice, although the timing of the sleep was altered, particularly in the m*Per2* mutants, who showed an advance of the locomotor activity rhythm.[26] Identification of circadian gene mutations that underlie a sleep homeostatic phenotype, independent of or in addition to the circadian phenotype, further shows that these systems are intricately linked even in their genetic basis. The evidence in animal studies suggests that a similar genetic predisposition may be involved in the cause of sleep regulation by the circadian and sleep systems in humans.

Several studies have established a genetic basis for circadian rhythm disorders. There have been several familial cases of ASP,[13,27–29] a published report of familial DSP,[30] and a study of patients with DSP found that a family history was reported in 11 of 53 individuals,[31] demonstrating the heritability of these conditions. In all published pedigrees, the affected phenotype segregates in an autosomal dominant manner. The first finding linking a gene to ASP identified a mutation in the human *PER2* gene that caused this condition in several members of a large family.[13] Other cases of familial ASP, however, did not carry this mutation thereby demonstrating genetic heterogeneity for this circadian rhythm sleep phase disorder. Genetic analysis of another ASP family led to the discovery of a mutation in another circadian gene, *CKIδ*, which was linked to the phenotype.[29] More recently, this same group identified a mutation in the circadian repressor gene *DEC2*, which was found in 2 relatives of a small family who had extremely early wake times.[32] In this case, however, the affected individuals did not have early bedtimes, as seen in most cases of ASP, and instead seem to be natural short sleepers. When this human mutation was expressed in both mouse and *Drosophila* models, this resulted in short sleep duration in these species. Furthermore, there was a marked reduction in recovery sleep after sleep deprivation in mice expressing this mutation compared with wildtype littermates, which indicates altered sleep homeostasis in the *DEC2* mutant. Thus, *DEC2* plays an important role in sleep regulation.

Genetic studies of idiopathic cases of DSP have also identified mutations in circadian genes that are associated with the delayed sleep phase phenotype. A haplotype of several mutations in the *PER3* gene was associated with cases of DSP in patients but not in controls.[33] A variable length polymorphism of the same gene, one of the mutations included in the haplotype, was found to associate with DSP and evening preference in a separate study.[34] A missense mutation in another circadian gene, the *CKIε* gene, was inversely associated with DSP and non–24-hour sleep/wake disorder.[35] Genetic analysis of circadian genes and their association with diurnal preference has revealed several gene variants that play a role in the regulation and timing of sleep in humans. An association between a polymorphism in the *CLOCK* gene and evening preference has been reported[36,37]; however, some studies have not show this same result.[38–40] Association studies have also identified polymorphisms in *PER1*[41] and *PER2*[42] genes that correlated with extreme diurnal preference.

SUMMARY

Circadian rhythm sleep phase disorders characterized by an altered phase timing of sleep affect a small but growing segment of the population. The study of these conditions may lead to discovery of the underlying mechanisms and therefore provide better treatment for alleviating the complaints and symptoms associated with them. Furthermore, the investigation of these disorders provides valuable insight into basic circadian physiologic regulation and interactions with various neurologic processes. Thorough phenotypic characterization of the circadian properties in patients with DSP and ASP may serve to elucidate critical pathways of light entrainment, and investigations of sleep in these individuals may reveal important mechanisms of the homeostatic processes affecting sleep and sleep timing. As technology advances, genetic analysis of circadian rhythm sleep disorders is likely to continue identifying genetic variants that modify the timing of sleep, as well as other chronobiological functions. Given the presence of circadian genes in multiple tissues, it is likely that identification of variants will uncover novel functions that go beyond circadian rhythms or sleep. Combining the tools of genetics with improved clinical diagnostic criteria and phenotypic evaluation will likely lead to greater understanding of the molecular and cellular mechanisms generating and regulating these complex processes. This may ultimately advance the treatment of circadian disorders to improve sleep, performance, and general health.

REFERENCES

1. American Academy of Sleep Medicine. The international classification of sleep disorders; diagnostic and coding manual. Westchester (IL): American Academy of Sleep Medicine; 2005.
2. Weitzman ED, Czeisler CA, Coleman RM, et al. Delayed sleep phase syndrome: a chronobiological disorder associated with sleep onset insomnia. Arch Gen Psychiatry 1981;38:737–46.
3. Uchiyama M, Okawa M, Shibui K, et al. Altered phase relation between sleep timing and core body temperature rhythm in delayed sleep phase syndrome and non-24-hour sleep-wake syndrome in humans. Neurosci Lett 2000;29:4101–4.
4. Schrader H, Bovim G, Sand T. The prevalence of delayed and advanced sleep phase syndromes. J Sleep Res 1993;2:51–5.
5. Yazaki M, Shirakawa S, Okawa M, et al. Demography of sleep disturbances associated with circadian rhythm disorders in Japan. Psychiatry Clin Neurosci 1999;53:267–8.
6. Kripke DF, Rex KM, Ancoli-Israel S, et al. Delayed sleep phase cases and controls. J Circadian Rhythms 2008;6:6.
7. Crowley SJ, Acebo C, Carskadon MA. Sleep, circadian rhythms, and delayed phase in adolescence. Sleep Med 2007;8:602–12.
8. Hazama GI, Inoue Y, Kojima K, et al. The prevalence of probable delayed-sleep-phase syndrome in students from junior high school to university in Tottori, Japan. Tohoku J Exp Med 2008;216:95–8.
9. Wolfson AR, Carskadon MA. Sleep schedules and daytime functioning in adolescents. Child Dev 1998;69:875–87.
10. Urner M, Tornic J, Bloch KE. Sleep patterns in high school and university students: a longitudinal study. Chronobiol Int 2009;26:1222–34.
11. Sadeh A, Dahl RE, Shahar G, et al. Sleep and the transition to adolescence: a longitudinal study. Sleep 2009;32:1602–9.
12. Dijk DJ, Duffy JF, Czeisler CA. Contribution of circadian physiology and sleep homeostasis to age-related changes in human sleep. Chronobiol Int 2000;17:285–311.
13. Jones CR, Campbell SS, Zone SE, et al. Familial advanced sleep-phase syndrome: a short-period circadian rhythm variant in humans. Nat Med 1999; 5:1062–5.
14. Ozaki S, Uchiyama M, Shirakawa S, et al. Prolonged interval from body temperature nadir to sleep offset in patients with delayed sleep phase syndrome. Sleep 1996;19:36–40.
15. Aoki H, Ozeki Y, Yamada N. Hypersensitivity of melatonin suppression in response to light in patients with delayed sleep phase syndrome. Chronobiol Int 2001;18:263–71.
16. Alvarez B, Dahlitz MJ, Vignau J, et al. The delayed sleep phase syndrome: clinical and investigative findings in 14 subjects. J Neurol Neurosurg Psychiatry 1992;55:665–70.
17. Uchiyama M, Okawa M, Shirakawa S, et al. A polysomnographic study on patients with delayed sleep phase syndrome (DSPS). Jpn J Psychiatry Neurol 1992;46:219–21.
18. Watanabe T, Kajimura N, Kato M, et al. Sleep and circadian rhythm disturbances in patients with delayed sleep phase syndrome. Sleep 2003;26:657–61.
19. Rahman SA, Kayumov L, Tchmoutina EA, et al. Clinical efficacy of dim light melatonin onset testing in diagnosing delayed sleep phase syndrome. Sleep Med 2009;10:549–55.
20. Uchiyama M, Okawa M, Shibui K, et al. Poor compensatory function for sleep loss as a pathogenic factor in patients with delayed sleep phase syndrome. Sleep 2000;23:553–8.
21. Mongrain V, Carrier J, Dumont M. Circadian and homeostatic sleep regulation in morningness-eveningness. J Sleep Res 2006;15:162–6.
22. Antoch MP, Song E-J, Chang A-M, et al. Functional identification of the mouse circadian clock gene by transgenic BAC rescue. Cell 1997;89:655–67.
23. King DP, Zhao Y, Sangoram AM, et al. Positional cloning of the mouse circadian clock gene. Cell 1997;89:641–53.
24. Naylor E, Bergmann BM, Krauski K, et al. The circadian Clock mutation alters sleep homeostasis in the mouse. J Neurosci 2000;20:8138–43.
25. Wisor JP, O'Hara BF, Terao A, et al. A role for cryptochromes in sleep regulation. BMC Neurosci 2002; 3:20.
26. Kopp C, Albrecht U, Zheng B, et al. Homeostatic sleep regulation is preserved in mPer1 and mPer2 mutant mice. Eur J Neurosci 2002;16:1099–106.
27. Reid KJ, Chang A-M, Dubocovich ML, et al. Familial advanced sleep phase syndrome. Arch Neurol 2001;58:1089–94.
28. Satoh K, Mishima K, Inoue Y, et al. Two pedigrees of familial advanced sleep phase syndrome in Japan. Sleep 2003;26:416–7.

29. Xu Y, Padiath QS, Shapiro RE, et al. Functional consequences of a CKIdelta mutation causing familial advanced sleep phase syndrome. Nature 2005;434:640–4.

30. Ancoli-Israel S, Schnierow B, Kelsoe J, et al. A pedigree of one family with delayed sleep phase syndrome. Chronobiol Int 2001;18:831–40.

31. Takahashi Y, Hohjoh H, Matsuura K. Predisposing factors in delayed sleep phase syndrome. Psychiatry Clin Neurosci 2000;54:356–8.

32. Vassalli A, Dijk DJ. Sleep function: current questions and new approaches. Eur J Neurosci 2009;29: 1830–41.

33. Ebisawa T, Uchiyama M, Kajimura N, et al. Association of structural polymorphisms in the human *period3* gene with delayed sleep phase syndrome. EMBO J 2001;2:342–6.

34. Archer SN, Robilliard DL, Skene DJ, et al. A length polymorphism in the circadian clock gene *Per3* is linked to delayed sleep phase syndrome and extreme diurnal preference. Sleep 2003;26:413–5.

35. Takano A, Uchiyama M, Kajimura N, et al. A missense variation in human casein kinase I epsilon gene that induces functional alteration and shows an inverse association with circadian rhythm sleep disorders. Neuropsychopharmacology 2004; 29:1901–9.

36. Katzenberg D, Young T, Finn L, et al. A clock polymorphism associated with human diurnal preference. Sleep 1998;21:569–76.

37. Mishima K, Tozawa T, Satoh K, et al. The 3111T/C polymorphism of hClock is associated with evening preference and delayed sleep timing in a Japanese population sample. Am J Med Genet B Neuropsychiatr Genet 2005;133:101–4.

38. Robilliard DL, Archer SN, Arendt J, et al. The 3111 clock gene polymorphism is not associated with sleep and circadian rhythmicity in phenotypically characterized human subjects. J Sleep Res 2002;11:305–12.

39. Johansson C, Willeit M, Smedh C, et al. Circadian clock-related polymorphisms in seasonal affective disorder and their relevance to diurnal preference. Neuropsychopharmacology 2003;28:734–9.

40. Pedrazzoli M, Louzada FM, Pereira DS, et al. Clock polymorphisms and circadian rhythms phenotypes in a sample of the Brazilian population. Chronobiol Int 2007;24:1–8.

41. Carpen JD, von schantz M, Smits M, et al. A silent polymorphism in the PER1 gene associates with extreme diurnal preference in humans. J Hum Genet 2006;51:1122–5.

42. Carpen JD, Archer SN, Skene DJ, et al. A single-nucleotide polymorphism in the 5'-untranslated region of the *hPER2* gene is associated with diurnal preference. J Sleep Res 2005;14:293–7.

Genetics of Insomnia

Philip R. Gehrman, PhD, CBSM[a],*, Enda Byrne, PhD[b],
Nathan Gillespie, PhD[c], Nicholas G. Martin, PhD[b]

KEYWORDS

• Insomnia • Insomnia-related genes • Heritability • Sleep

Despite insomnia being the most common sleep disorder, little is known about the contribution of genetics to its etiology and pathophysiology. Between 6% and 10% of individuals experience insomnia that is chronic in nature, whereas another 25% report occasional difficulties with sleep.[1] Insomnia is also associated with several negative sequelae including fatigue, irritability, and impaired concentration and memory. Longitudinal studies have also repeatedly shown that insomnia is a risk factor for the development of new-onset mood, anxiety, and substance-use disorders.[2] Given the prevalence of insomnia and its associated public health impact, advances in our understanding of the genetic underpinnings of the disorder could lead to prevention and treatment efforts that would benefit a substantial proportion of the population. The goal of this review is to provide an overview of the current literature on the genetics of insomnia and to propose a research agenda for future studies.

WHAT IS THE INSOMNIA PHENOTYPE?

As in all genetics studies, a critical issue is the manner in which the insomnia phenotype is defined. Insomnia research has long been plagued by widely varying phenotypic definitions used in both genetic and nongenetic studies that have hampered attempts to synthesize the literature. Efforts have been made to create more standardized assessment approaches and definitions,[3,4] but substantial heterogeneity continues.

At the most fundamental level, insomnia can be assessed with the single question, "Do you have trouble sleeping?" While this question has apparent surface validity, it is associated with several difficulties including individual differences in beliefs about what constitutes "trouble," introducing a variable threshold for reporting difficulty. The variability lies in the severity (eg, how many minutes it takes to fall asleep), frequency (ie, how many nights per week), and duration (ie, how many weeks/months/ years) of the insomnia. If a low threshold is chosen, the lifetime prevalence of insomnia would likely be close to 100% given that an occasional night of difficulty sleeping is a nearly ubiquitous phenomenon. In research studies, common thresholds that are used are:

- Severity: $\geq$30 minutes sleep-onset latency (SOL; the time it takes to fall asleep) and/or $\geq$30 minutes of wake after sleep onset (WASO; the amount of time spent awake during the night) and/or $\geq$30 minutes early-morning awakening (EMA; the time between actual and desired wake-up times)
- Frequency: 3 or more nights per week
- Duration: >1 month (>6 months for some studies).

An advantage of criteria such as these is that they permit both categorical and dimensional distinctions to be made.

Current clinical[5,6] and research[4] diagnostic systems do not include these thresholds, but they do require that the insomnia be associated with some degree of associated distress or

[a] Department of Psychiatry, University of Pennsylvania, 3535 Market Street, Suite 670, Philadelphia, PA 19104, USA
[b] Psychiatric Genetics, Queensland Institute of Medical Research, 300 Herston Road, Brisbane, QLD 4029, Australia
[c] Department of Psychiatry, Virginia Institute for Psychiatric and Behavior Genetics, Virginia Commonwealth University, 800 East Leigh Street, Biotech 1, Suite 101, Richmond, VA 23219-1534, USA
* Corresponding author.
E-mail address: gehrman@exchange.upenn.edu

Sleep Med Clin 6 (2011) 191–202
doi:10.1016/j.jsmc.2011.03.003
1556-407X/11/$ – see front matter. Published by Elsevier Inc.

impairment. In clinical settings this requirement is almost always met because an individual is not likely to seek treatment for insomnia if he or she does not perceive it to be causing negative consequences. In studies of community samples there is consistently a portion of the population that reports difficulty initiating or maintaining sleep, but that does not report associated consequences.[7] The necessity of the distress or impairment criterion is clear for clinical settings, but its applicability for genetic studies is less certain. Current diagnostic systems also divide insomnia into several specific subtypes including psychophysiologic, idiopathic, and paradoxic forms that reflect the presumed heterogeneity of this patient population. Some studies have also focused on the distinctions among sleep onset (early), sleep maintenance (middle), and early-morning awakening (late) subtypes. As with psychiatric disorders, diagnostic subtypes are based on observable distinctions among groups of patients rather than underlying etiologic dimensions, so it is not known whether genetic studies should use these categories.

The phenotypic considerations reviewed thus far rely on subjective, self-report assessment methods and are therefore susceptible to perceptual and cognitive biases. For example, isolated "bad" nights of sleep may be particularly salient and influence retrospective judgments of sleep made about a period of time that actually included a higher frequency of "good" nights. Subjective estimates of sleep also have the inherent limitation of requiring the respondent to perceive a state of reduced consciousness and awareness. It is well established that self-reports of physical symptoms are influenced by several other factors including current depression and anxiety, sociocultural beliefs, and individual differences in "body awareness," among others.[8] Investigations of the pathophysiology of insomnia that rely on self-report measures need to consider the possibility that findings are associated with these broader self-report influences rather than insomnia per se.

Objective measures of sleep have the potential to eliminate the factors associated with self-reported insomnia. The gold standard for the objective measurement of sleep is polysomnography (PSG), which involves the simultaneous measurement of electroencephalographic (EEG), electromyographic, and electrooculographic activity at a minimum, with the potential to acquire several other biologic signals. Traditionally, PSG data are scored according to standard rules to determine which stage of sleep (1, 2, 3, 4, or rapid eye movement [REM]) best characterizes a period of data and the subsequent computation of sleep architecture

parameters. As reviewed by Watson elsewhere in this issue, sleep architectural variables appear to represent individual traits that are highly heritable, suggesting that PSG may be an optimal strategy for genetics studies of insomnia. A practical limitation is that PSG is time consuming and expensive, limiting its applicability for most large-scale studies. A larger issue is that several PSG studies have failed to find objective evidence of disturbed sleep in individuals with subjective reports of insomnia. This discrepancy remained an enigma until it was realized that there may be inherent limitations in using visual methods for determining sleep and wake, given that EEG signals contain a level of complexity that may require more sophisticated analysis methods.

A growing number of studies have now used computer-based spectral analysis methods to provide a finer-grained analysis of the microarchitecture of sleep. Individuals with insomnia, compared with good sleepers, frequently demonstrate increased EEG activity in the beta frequency range during visually determined sleep.[9] Beta EEG is usually seen during periods of waking mental activity rather than sleep, leading to the hypothesis that insomnia can be associated with a "mixed" state of wakefulness and sleep that is perceived as wakefulness by the individual. This proposal would explain the discrepancy between subjective and objective assessments of sleep found in many insomnia studies. Sleep architectural and microarchitectural features thus offer potential phenotypes for genetic studies of insomnia.

IS INSOMNIA A HERITABLE TRAIT?

A necessary initial step in studying the genetics of insomnia is to establish that it is indeed a trait that is influenced by genetic factors. In studying the genetic influence on phenotypic traits, it is usual to estimate heritability in the narrow sense (h^2), that is, the proportion of variation in the trait that can be explained by additive genetic factors. The two strategies most frequently used to establish heritability are twin and family studies.

Twin Studies

In studies of monozygotic (MZ) and dizygotic (DZ) twins reared together who have 100% and approximately 50% of their genes in common, respectively, phenotypic variation can be decomposed and explained by additive genetic (A), common environment (C), and random environment (E) variance components.[10,11] Several twin studies have investigated the genetic and environmental etiology of insomnia phenotypes (summarized in **Table 1**). The first of these was

Table 1
Twin studies of insomnia phenotypes

Authors, Ref. Year	Sample	Phenotypes	Heritability
Webb and Campbell,[12] 1983	14 MZ, 14 DZ Young adults	Sleep latency Wake time	No data available
Partinen et al,[13] 1983	2238 MZ, 4545 DZ Adults	Sleep length Sleep quality	$h^2 = 0.44$ $h^2 = 0.44$
Heath et al,[14] 1990	1792 MZ, 2101 DZ Adults	Sleep quality Initial insomnia Sleep latency Anxious insomnia Depressed insomnia	$h^2 = 0.32$ $h^2 = 0.32$ $h^2 = 0.44 \, \male, 0.32 \, \female$ $h^2 = 0.36$ $h^2 = 0.33$
Heath et al,[15] 1998	1792 MZ, 2101 DZ Adults	Composite score	12.1% of variance in ♀, 8.3% in ♂
McCarren et al,[16] 1994	1605 MZ, 1200 DZ Male veterans	Trouble falling asleep Trouble staying asleep Waking up several times Waking up tired Composite score	$h^2 = 0.28$ $h^2 = 0.42$ $h^2 = 0.26$ $h^2 = 0.21$ $h^2 = 0.28$
De Castro,[17] 2002	86 MZ, 129 DZ Adult "good sleepers"	Sleep duration No. of wakeups	$h^2 = 0.30$ $h^2 = 0.21$
Watson et al,[18] 2006	1042 MZ, 828 DZ Young adults	Insomnia	$h^2 = 0.64$
Boomsma et al,[19] 2008	548 twins, 265 siblings Adults	Insomnia factor	$h^2 = 0.20$
Gregory et al,[20] 2004	2162 MZ, 4229 DZ Age 3–7 y	Sleep problems scale	$h^2 = 0.18 \, \male, 0.20 \, \female$
Gregory et al,[21,23] 2006	100 MZ, 200 DZ Age 8 y	Sleep onset delay Night wakings	$h^2 = 0.17$ for child report, 0.79 for parental report $h^2 = 0.27$ for child report, 0.32 for parental report
Gregory,[22] 2008	100 MZ, 200 DZ Age 8 y	Dyssomnia scale	$h^2 = 0.71$
Gregory et al,[21,23] 2006	192 MZ, 384 DZ Age 8 y	Sleep problems score	$h^2 = 0.61$

conducted by Webb and Campbell,[12] who studied 14 MZ and 14 DZ twin pairs. Their sample consisted of self-defined good sleepers who underwent one night of PSG. Although the participants did not have insomnia, the study is relevant in that there were significant dominant genetic effects for both SOL and several measures of time spent awake during the night. It is likely that these sleep characteristics are normally distributed in the population, with those individuals at one extreme reporting insomnia. In the same year, Partinen and colleagues[13] collected self-reported sleep data from a much larger sample of 2238 MZ and 4545 DZ adult twin pairs with greater power to detect genetic and environmental components of variance, and found significant

heritability for sleep length ($h^2 = 0.44$) and sleep quality ($h^2 = 0.44$). Both sleep length and sleep quality are phenotypes representing broad constructs that nevertheless have some relevance for insomnia.

The twin study with the broadest assessment of sleep and insomnia phenotypes to date was conducted with the Australian twin registry and was reported by Heath and colleagues.[14] Their survey of 1792 MZ and 2101 DZ twin pairs included several questions related to sleep quality, disturbance, and overall patterns. Of most relevance for insomnia, additive genetic influences were found for sleep quality ($h^2 = 0.32$), initial insomnia ($h^2 = 0.32$), SOL ($h^2 = 0.44$ for men and 0.32 for women), "anxious insomnia" ($h^2 = 0.36$), and "depressed insomnia" ($h^2 = 0.33$). SOL was the only variable for which there were significant gender effects. Follow-up analyses were reported in a second article that used a very different statistical approach to examine heritability.[15] A composite sleep disturbance factor was computed and used as the dependent variable in regression analyses, which indicated that genetic influences accounted for 12.1% of the variance in the sleep disturbance factor for females and 8.3% for males. After controlling for anxiety, depression, and neuroticism, there were still significant genetic effects over and above these influences. These values cannot be directly compared with heritability estimates reported in other studies, because of the different analytical approach employed.

McCarren and colleagues[16] studied 1605 MZ and 1200 DZ male twin pairs from the Vietnam Era Twin Registry, asking about several aspects of sleep, which were examined separately and as a composite score. Heritability estimates for each measure were: trouble falling asleep ($h^2 = 0.28$), trouble staying asleep ($h^2 = 0.42$), waking up several times per night ($h^2 = 0.26$), waking up feeling tired and worn out ($h^2 = 0.21$), and the composite sleep score ($h^2 = 0.28$). A study of sleep patterns in a small study based on 86 MZ and 129 DZ "good sleeper" twins reared together from the Minnesota Twin Registry examined the genetic contributions to 1-week sleep diary variables of sleep duration, wake duration, sleep latency, and number of wake-ups.[17] Heritability of the sleep parameters ranged from 0.21 to 0.41, although there was no evidence of significant genetic influences on SOL. Watson and colleagues[18] surveyed 1042 MZ and 828 DZ twins from the Washington State twin registry. A single item on insomnia was included, which had a heritability of 0.64. In a survey of 548 twins and 265 siblings, Boomsma and colleagues[19] administered the Dutch Groningen Sleep Questionnaire. Principal-components analysis found that the insomnia-related questions clustered on a single factor, which had a heritability of 0.20.

Several studies have been conducted by Gregory and colleagues[20] examining sleep problems in youth. In their first study, 6000 twin pairs completed a survey that contained a 4-item "sleep problem" scale related to "hard to get to sleep," "frequent wakings," "nightmares," and "early waking." Total scores on this scale showed modest evidence of additive genetic influence ($h^2 = 0.18$ for boys and 0.20 for girls). A second study of 300 8-year-old twin pairs involved both parental ratings of their child's sleep and the child's self-ratings of their sleep.[21] Parents and children used different, but highly similar, validated

sleep questionnaires each containing 8 subscales related to various aspects of disturbed sleep in children, with the "sleep onset delay" and "night wakings" subscales having greatest relevance as insomnia phenotypes. Estimates of additive genetic influences on the sleep-onset delay subscale were very different for parental ($h^2 = 0.79$) as compared with child ($h^2 = 0.17$) ratings. Estimates for the night wakings subscale were more comparable, with estimates of 0.32 and 0.27 for parental and child reports, respectively. In a reanalysis of these data a "dyssomnia" scale was computed based on 10 items from the parental rating scale, most of which are of relevance for insomnia (eg, sleep-onset delay and sleep duration).[22] Total scores on the dyssomnia scale showed evidence of substantial heritability ($h^2 = 0.71$). A second cohort of 300 8-year-old twin pairs was selected on the basis of having either high or low anxiety ratings.[23] Using the same parental sleep rating scale, a "sleep problems" score was computed that was found to be highly heritable ($h^2 = 0.61$). These children were reassessed 2 years later (at age 10), when almost an identical estimate ($h^2 = 0.63$) was found.[24]

Taken together, these twin studies demonstrate that insomnia-related phenotypes consistently demonstrate evidence that genes play an etiologic role, with primarily additive effects. With only a few exceptions, heritability estimates in adults were consistently in the range of 0.25 to 0.45, regardless of the exact question or phenotype used. In children, parental estimates of "sleep problems" demonstrate substantially greater heritability, with estimates across studies ranging from 0.60 to 0.80. Of importance, the study that contained both parental and child sleep[21] ratings found lower heritability estimates when the children rated their own sleep. It may be that mild sleep problems are more likely to go unnoticed by parents, so that their ratings capture mostly the more severe cases. Alternatively, youth may have poorer understanding of the questionnaire items, which could increase the error variance. More severe sleep problems may have stronger genetic underpinnings than when the full spectrum of severity is considered together. Twin studies thus indicate that insomnia, broadly defined, is moderately heritable when rated by the individual, with approximately one-third of the variance in symptoms attributable to genetic factors.

Family History Studies

An alternative approach to demonstrating the influence of genetic factors is the family history approach. In family history studies, family members of individuals affected with the condition of interest are compared with family members of unaffected individuals. If genetic factors contribute to the condition, the family members of affected individuals will be more likely to also report the condition than those of unaffected individuals. Only 6 family history studies of insomnia have been conducted.

In an early study, Abe and Shimakawa[25] compared the sleep patterns of parents with their 3-year-old children. Parents who reported sleeping poorly as children, in terms of the depth of their sleep and the ease of falling asleep, tended to have children who also reported similar patterns. Though somewhat crude in its methodological approach, this study demonstrates that the notion that insomnia tends to run in families is not new.

In one of the only studies of childhood-onset insomnia, Hauri and Olmstead[26] compared individuals whose insomnia originated in childhood with those with adult-onset difficulties. Both groups tended to report a family history of sleep complaints, but this rate was higher in the childhood-onset (55%) than in the adult-onset (39%) group. In a study of patients in a sleep disorders clinic, 35% of those with insomnia reported one or more family members also experiencing some form of sleep disturbance, of which the most common form reported was insomnia.[27] In support of the Hauri study, there was trend toward higher rates in the families of those with an earlier age of onset. The same group recruited a second clinic sample of 181 patients with insomnia, this time also recruiting a control group without insomnia.[28] Patients were classified into the diagnostic subtypes of primary insomnia or psychiatric insomnia. There was a positive family history of insomnia in 72.7% of individuals with primary insomnia, 43.4% of those with psychiatric insomnia, and 24.1% of controls.

Beaulieu-Bonneau and colleagues[29] surveyed approximately 1000 individuals and categorized them as good sleepers (52.0%), having symptoms of insomnia (32.5%), and meeting criteria for a full insomnia syndrome (15.5%). There was a positive family history of insomnia in these groups of 32.7%, 36.7%, and 38.1%, respectively, with no significant group differences in these rates. However, in further analysis they divided the good sleepers into those with and without a personal history of insomnia, and found that those without a personal history had a significantly lower rate of family history (29.0%) than those with a personal history (48.9%). This finding highlights a difficulty of studying insomnia, a disorder whose clinical state can vary over time such that individuals who are good sleepers at the time of

assessment may have a prior history of insomnia, thus making it unclear whether they are truly controls.

One last study deserves mention in its use of a novel insomnia phenotype. As mentioned previously, a difficulty in identifying an insomnia case is that the sleep difficulty can vary over time, with periods of relatively good sleep and periods of insomnia. Depending on when an individual is assessed, they could be classified as either an individual with insomnia or a good sleeper. Drake and colleagues[30] created a scale called the Ford Insomnia Response to Stress Test (FIRST) that attempts to measure an individual's vulnerability to experience disturbed sleep in response to a stressor. The FIRST avoids the problems associated with measuring current sleep quantity and quality by assessing the trait measure of insomnia vulnerability, with higher scores indicating greater vulnerability. A small family history study has been conducted with the FIRST, in which it was administered to 31 sibling pairs.[31] The within-pair correlation was 0.61, indicating that 37.2% of the variance in FIRST scores is attributable to familial aggregation. Future work is needed to determine whether the FIRST will be a useful phenotype for studying the genetics of insomnia.

The small body of family history studies of insomnia is in agreement with the twin studies in demonstrating a modest degree of genetic influences. Although further work is needed to better understand the genetic contributions to various insomnia phenotypes, there is a sufficient base of evidence to pursue studies to identify which genes are related to insomnia.

GENES RELATED TO INSOMNIA

Two general approaches can be used to identify genes related to insomnia. In the first approach, candidate genes can be selected for investigation based on known mechanisms of sleep-wake regulation. Alternatively, gene discovery strategies such as linkage and genome-wide association studies (GWAS) can recruit individuals with an insomnia phenotype, defined either categorically or as a quantitative dimension, to search for genes that are systematically related to the phenotype. Very few discovery studies have been conducted to date.

Candidate Gene Approaches

A great deal is known about the neural mechanisms involved in sleep-wake regulation. As such, an alternative to gene discovery approaches is to identify candidate genes that may affect insomnia based on their known role in the neural systems that affect sleep. A logical place to start is with the genes involved in the generation of circadian rhythms, given the role that they play in sleep-wake regulation. These so-called clock genes have been well characterized, as have the transcriptional-translational feedback loops through which these genes produce an oscillatory system.[32] Several studies have examined the relationships among sleep-wake characteristics and clock genes, which may be of relevance for insomnia.

Laposky and colleagues[33] created mice carrying a null allele for the BMAL1/Mop3 gene. These mice demonstrated alterations in circadian rhythms, as would be expected, but they also had alterations in sleep-wake characteristics including more fragmentation of sleep, reduced duration of sleep bouts, and altered total sleep time. In human studies, Viola and colleagues[34] focused on the *PER3* gene, and compared individuals homozygous for either the short (*PER3^{4/4}*) or long (*PER3^{5/5}*) alleles. The group with the long allele had a shorter SOL and spent a greater proportion of the night in slow-wave sleep than the short allele group. Of note, several studies have examined the relationships between clock genes and sleep homeostasis, which may be relevant for the study of insomnia. The reader is referred to the article by Goel elsewhere in this issue for a review of these studies.

In one group of studies, the relationships between clock genes and sleep-wake characteristics have been studied in the context of mood disorders. Sleep is frequently disturbed in patients with mood disorders, and several studies have now found evidence that clock genes are associated with mood disorder diagnoses.[35] For example, Serretti and colleagues[36] found an association between 3111T/C *CLOCK* gene polymorphisms and insomnia symptoms in a large cohort of patients with major depressive disorder. The TC and CC genotypes were associated with higher rates of sleep onset and sleep maintenance insomnia, as well as early-morning awakenings. The same group reported in a second cohort of that the C variant was not associated with baseline insomnia in a mixed group of mood disorders patients, but that it was related to development of insomnia during treatment with selective serotonin reuptake inhibitors.[37] In a larger cohort study in Finland, Utge and colleagues[38] examined the associations between 113 single-nucleotide polymorphisms (SNPs) across 18 clock genes and sleep disturbance in individuals with depression and controls. The investigators found that the *TIMELESS* gene was associated with early-morning awakenings in the depressed group, but that this effect was different for men and women.

These studies indicate that studying a patient population known to experience sleep disturbance may be a fruitful approach to identifying genes of relevance for insomnia.

In addition to the clock genes, several studies have examined genes related to the various neurotransmitter systems involved in sleep-wake regulation. The findings of these studies have implications for the genetics of insomnia.

Serotonin

One of the most frequently studied genes is that for the serotonin transporter polymorphic region (5HTTLPR). The short allele is associated with reduced efficiency of transcription and has been shown to be a risk factor for several psychiatric disorders. It is not surprising that this gene has also been examined in relation to insomnia phenotypes. In a small pharmacogenetic study of patients with major depressive disorder, the short allele was associated with an increased likelihood of developing new or worsening insomnia in response to fluoxetine treatment.[39] Brummett and colleagues[40] examined the relationship between 5HTTLPR genotype and sleep quality in caregivers of individuals with dementia and non-caregiver controls. There was no significant main effect of genotype on sleep quality, but there was a significant gene × environment interaction with caregiving such that individuals with the short allele who were caregivers were more likely to report poor sleep quality than those with the long allele, but there was no relationship for non-caregivers. Kang and colleagues[41] examined the influence of the serotonin receptor 2A gene −1438A/G polymorphisms on the impact of mirtazapine treatment on sleep in patients with major depressive disorder. The G/G genotype was associated with less improvement in sleep with treatment as compared with carriers of the A+ allele. The availability of serotonin (and other monoamines) in the brain is in part regulated by monoamine oxidase A (MAO-A), so 2 studies have examined the relationships between MAO-A polymorphisms and sleep characteristics. Brummett and colleagues[42] found that the low-activity (3-repeat) allele was associated with poorer sleep compared with higher-activity alleles (3.5-repeat and 4-repeat). By contrast, Craig and colleagues[43] found that the 4-repeat allele conferred the greatest risk of sleep disruption in a sample of patients with Alzheimer disease.

Dopamine

Two animal studies have examined the effects of knockout of the dopamine transporter (DAT). The first study, conducted in mice, found that

DAT knockouts had reduced non-REM sleep time and shorter duration of sleep bouts on average.[44] In flies, DAT knockouts displayed reduced sleep time and increased wakefulness.[45] These studies provide additional evidence that dopamine does plays a role in sleep-wake regulation. Although somewhat speculative, one could hypothesize that excessive dopamine activity may bias the sleep-wake system toward increased wakefulness at night and increase the risk for insomnia.

γ-Aminobutyric acid

With only one exception, the mechanism of action of hypnotic medications is through the inhibitory γ-aminobutyric acid (GABA) system. As such it would be logical to expect that genes that affect GABA neurotransmission would affect sleep. Buhr and colleagues[46] reported a case study of a patient with a missense mutation of the β3 subunit of the GABA$_A$ receptor. The patient had insomnia, as did several members of his family, suggesting that this mutation may have affected their sleep. Agosto and colleagues[47] examined *Drosophila* with the mutant GABA$_A$ receptor *Rdl*^{A302S}, which is associated with increased channel current. Flies with this mutant receptor exhibited decreased SOL.

Adenosine

Adenosine is thought to play a role in the regulation of sleep homeostasis. Adenosine receptors are also likely the site of action of caffeine. Therefore genes affecting adenosine activity in the brain could be of relevance to insomnia. Retey and colleagues[48] examined the relationship between adenosine deaminase gene polymorphisms and sleep laboratory measures. Individuals with the G/A allele had fewer awakenings at night, spent more time in slow-wave sleep, and had higher delta power than those with the G/G allele. In a second study by the same group a relationship was found between the adenosine A$_{2A}$ receptor gene (*ADOR-A2A*) and individual response to caffeine, whereby the C/C genotype was more common in caffeine-sensitive subjects.[49] This result is replicated in the Australian twin cohort mentioned previously (E. Byrne, unpublished data, 2010). The report also contained the results of an Internet survey in which insomnia symptoms were found to be more prevalent in caffeine-sensitive subjects, providing an indirect link between adenosine receptor polymorphisms and insomnia phenotypes. Lastly, Gass and colleagues[50] focused on 117 SNPs from 13 genes related to adenosine transporters, receptors, and metabolism enzymes in cases with depression and controls. Polymorphisms in the *SLC29A3* gene, related to adenosine metabolism, were associated with depression involving early-morning awakenings in women. In men there was a suggestive association of *SLC28A1* and depression with early-morning awakenings. These studies provide preliminary evidence that adenosine-related genes may relate to insomnia phenotypes, directly or as mediated through sleep homeostatic mechanisms.

Hypocretin/orexin

There has been an increased interest in recent years in the role that hypocretins/orexins play in sleep regulation. Prober and colleagues[51] created zebrafish that overexpressed hypocretin. This fish produces a phenotype characterized by hyperarousal and reduced ability to initiate and maintain sleep. The investigators hypothesize that this phenotype is akin to insomnia.

Other candidate genes

One final study relevant to the genetics of insomnia was conducted by Liu and colleagues,[52] who studied mutation of the *amnesiac* gene in *Drosophila*, which is related to protein kinase A activity. Flies with a mutation in *amnesiac* had fragmented sleep and shortened sleep latency. The investigators suggest that this gene is involved in the regulation of sleep onset and maintenance.

In summary, these candidate gene studies indicate that genes affecting a wide array of neural processes may have some bearing on insomnia phenotypes. As is the case in all candidate gene studies, replication will be essential before any conclusions can be drawn. Given the sheer number of potential genetic influences, a great deal of work will be needed to better understand how these and related genes interact to produce insomnia phenotypes.

Gene Discovery Studies

The first gene discovery study of sleep-related phenotypes was reported by Gottlieb and colleagues[53] from a subset (n = 749) of the Framingham Heart Study Offspring Cohort. These investigators were not examining insomnia phenotypes, but their measures of usual bedtime and sleep duration are of some relevance. Linkage analysis failed to find any peaks with logarithm of odds (LOD) greater than 3, but 5 peaks with LOD greater than 2 were found, including a linkage between usual bedtime and *CSNK2A2*, a gene known to be a component of the circadian molecular clock. The data were then examined in population-based and family-based association tests. No results reached genome-wide significance, which is not surprising given the sample size, and of the results with the lowest P values only one was located in a coding region. Usual bedtime was associated with the SNP rs324981, located in the gene NPSR1, which is a component of the neuropeptide S receptor. While not a study of insomnia, this investigation is important in establishing the feasibility of finding genetic associations with self-reported sleep phenotypes.

A more recent linkage study examined the novel phenotype of sleep disturbance attributed to caffeine intake.[54] The feelings of wakefulness associated with caffeine intake are thought to be due to antagonism of the adenosine pathway, and hence variation in caffeine sensitivity may be due to genetic variants that also influence general sleep. Data were taken from the Australian twin registry previously cited as one of the first twin studies of insomnia phenotypes[14] in which follow-up genetic data (n = 1989) provided data for gene discovery analyses. As a first step, the various insomnia phenotypes were subjected to a Cholesky decomposition, which showed that coffee-attributed insomnia had unique genetic effects not shared with other insomnia phenotypes. Of note, a single factor loaded on all of the insomnia phenotypes, suggesting that genetic influences on insomnia may broadly affect several aspects of the disorder rather than being specific to particular characteristics. Linkage analysis found a significant relationship between coffee-attributed insomnia and a region on chromosome 2q (LOD = 2.9).

Animal models provide more opportunities for gene discovery studies, as they allow for experimental breeding and other approaches not possible in human studies. For example, Wu and colleagues[55] conducted a forward genetic screen in Drosophila of approximately 3000 lines to identify short-sleeping mutants. Short-sleeping flies tended to sleep in shorter bouts than longer-sleeping flies, suggesting that they may have had difficulty with sleep maintenance, an important insomnia phenotype. Of note, the number of sleep bouts was not reduced, indicating that sleep initiation was not impaired. It is interesting that the short-sleeping flies also exhibited reduced arousal thresholds and were more easily awoken. These phenotypic differences mapped to a novel allele of the dopamine transporter gene. It is not known whether these flies were short-sleepers because of impaired sleep ability (ie, insomnia) or reduced sleep need, but the reduced arousal threshold of these mutants suggests some degree of overlap with insomnia.

A different approach was taken by Seugnet and colleagues,[56] who selectively bred flies that exhibited shorter sleep durations. After 60 generations, they were able to produce flies they referred to as insomnia-like (ins-l) whose total sleep time was only 60 minutes per day. These flies further demonstrated difficulties both with initiating and maintaining sleep, increased activity levels during waking, and impairments in learning on an avoidance task and in motor coordination. The investigators propose that this animal model captures both the nighttime and daytime characteristics of insomnia. Gene profiling identified 1350 genes that were differentially expressed in the ins-l flies compared with wild-type flies, many of which fell into categories related to metabolism, neuronal activity, behavior, and sensory perception. The investigators argue that the phenotypes observed are due to the small effects of a large number of genes rather than large effects in a few genes, a hypothesis that is consistent with the results from large genetic association studies in humans.

Yet a different approach was taken by Winrow and colleagues,[57] who crossed 2 inbred mouse strains to create a large number of offspring (n = 269). For each mouse, sleep was recorded for 48 hours and used to compute 20 sleep-wake variables that reduced to 5 traits in a factor analysis: amount of sleep, sleep fragmentation, REM sleep traits, latency to REM or non-REM sleep, and relative EEG spectral power. These traits were then subjected to quantitative trait loci (QTL) analysis to identify genes associated with each of these traits. Linkage analysis identified 52 significant QTL associated with these traits with LOD scores ranging from 2.5 to 7.6.

This collection of studies is noteworthy in the degree to which they represent some of the various research strategies that can be used for discovery of genes that may relate to insomnia. It is also noteworthy that so few studies have been conducted, several of which involved phenotypes of only marginal significance for insomnia. A great deal of further work clearly needs to be done.

FUTURE DIRECTIONS FOR GENE DISCOVERY

The next step in the quest to find genetic variants that contribute to insomnia risk is to perform more refined GWAS, which permit testing for association between millions of common markers (>1% minor allele frequency) that span most of the human genome, and complex phenotypes. The advantage of this approach is that it requires no prior hypothesis about which genes are likely to influence the trait, and is instead considered to be hypothesis generating. On the other hand, performing millions of tests means that thousands of markers will be significantly associated with the trait simply by chance, therefore strict significance thresholds must be used to limit false-positive associations. GWAS has become feasible in the last few years because of the discovery that the human genome can be divided up into haplotype blocks, the common variation in which can be tagged by only a few polymorphic markers, combined with the gradual reduction in the cost of genotyping large numbers of markers accurately.

Since 2006, GWAS have been undertaken for a plethora of diseases and complex traits with varying degrees of success.[58] In many cases, the genes or pathways identified would not previously have been suspected as influencing the trait,[59] and genes known to be involved in other traits harbor variants that influence other seemingly unrelated traits. In other cases, loci previously known to harbor rare Mendelian mutations with large effects on the phenotype have also been found to carry variants with much smaller effect. A rare mutation in the low-density lipoprotein (LDL) receptor gene causes familial hypercholesterolemia, but other variants in the region have a weak effect on the level of LDL cholesterol.[60] GWAS of insomnia phenotypes may show that common variants in genes for rare Mendelian sleep disorders harbor common variants that influence insomnia.

The success of the GWAS approach has varied widely depending on the trait that has been analyzed. This variation is partly due to certain studies having larger sample sizes or more efficient study designs, but likely also reflects differing genetic architectures between traits.[61] As an example of these differing architectures, there have been 5 replicated associations for age-related macular degeneration that together explain 50% of the heritability of the disease,[62] whereas there have been 18 replicated associations for type 2 diabetes that together explain only 6% of the heritability.[63] By contrast, a recent study of serum-transferrin levels showed that a very small number of SNPs explain 40% of the heritability.[64] In the main, however, the effect sizes have been small, highlighting the need for large sample sizes to detect the signals.

Whether GWAS studies are successful in finding insomnia genes will be dependent on the genetic architecture underlying the particular insomnia phenotype under investigation and the sample sizes used in the study. The genetic architecture will depend on the forces of selection that have acted over time. In the main it appears that for most diseases, natural selection has acted to remove variants of large effect, and so the total genetic risk to disease is due to the cumulative effect of many variants, each of which explains only a small proportion of the overall genetic risk. Even for a quantitative trait such as height that is not associated with negative outcomes, it has been shown that common variants of very small effect explain almost 60% of the total phenotypic variance.[65] Given the importance of sleep for proper physiologic functioning and that insomnia is associated with several negative sequelae that reduce quality of life, one can speculate that many genes of small effect may also explain the heritability of insomnia. Highly penetrant genes would likely have been selected against. If the genetic architecture is such that there are many genes of small effect, then it will take very large sample sizes to detect associated variants.

As with all association studies, replication is the gold standard, and any genetic variants detected via the GWAS method will need to replicated in an independent sample. Because different groups collect phenotypic information on insomnia in different ways, replication may be difficult to achieve. One of the central issues in association studies is that of power, that is, given there is a real association between a marker and the trait, what are the chances that the study design will detect the association? If a study has only a small chance of detecting a true effect, then money and time may be wasted on a fruitless search. There are several factors that affect power: the heritability of the trait, the sample size, effect size of the causative allele, frequency of the causative allele, and, if the actual causative allele has not been typed, the degree of linkage disequilibrium (LD) between the causative SNP and a typed SNP. Power can vary depending on the study design, but in all cases the power to detect an association between a given SNP (S) and a causal variant (V) can be described as:

$$\text{Power} \ \alpha \ \left(r_{s,v}^2 \right) n q^2$$

where $r_{s,v}^2$ is the LD between the SNP and the causal variant, n is the sample size, and q^2 is the proportion of phenotypic variance explained by the causal variant.[66] If we assume there are no dominance effects attributable to the causal allele and the allele is in Hardy-Weinberg Equilibrium, then q^2 is given by:

$$q^2 = \frac{2p(1-p)a^2}{\sigma_p^2}$$

where a is the mean effect of the homozygote genotype of the causal allele, p is the allele frequency, and σ_p^2 is the total phenotypic variance.[67] From these equations it can be easily seen that the more variance in a trait that a genetic variant explains, the easier it will be to detect. As the explained variance is dependent on the allele frequency, focusing on common variants is desirable. The only parameter that the experimenter has control over is the sample size. For variants that explain only a small fraction of the variance, large sample sizes will be required for detection.

Our understanding of the genetics of insomnia, while primitive, points in several directions for future research. This area is ripe for studies that could shed light on the processes of both normal and pathologic sleep. The end result could be improved identification of individuals at risk and the development of novel treatments for insomnia.

REFERENCES

1. Ohayon MM. Epidemiology of insomnia: what we know and what we still need to learn. Sleep Med Rev 2002;6:97–111.
2. Ford D, Kamerow D. Epidemiologic study of sleep disturbance and psychiatric disorders: an opportunity for prevention? JAMA 1989;262:1479–84.
3. Buysse DJ, Ancoli-Israel S, Edinger JD, et al. Recommendations for a standard research assessment of insomnia. Sleep 2006;29:1155–73.
4. Edinger JD, Bonnet MH, Bootzin RR, et al. Derivation of research diagnostic criteria for insomnia: report of an American Academy of Sleep Medicine work group. Sleep 2004;27:1567–96.
5. American Psychiatric Association. Diagnostic and statistical manual of mental disorders. Text revision. 4th edition. Washington, DC: American Psychiatric Association; 2000.
6. American Academy of Sleep Medicine. International classification of sleep disorders. 2nd edition. Darien (IL): American Academy of Sleep Medicine; 2005.
7. Fichten CS, Creti L, Amsel R, et al. Poor sleepers who do not complain of insomnia: myths and realities about psychological and lifestyle characteristics of older good and poor sleepers. J Behav Med 1995;18:189–223.
8. Kolk AM, Hanewald GJ, Schagen S, et al. A symptom perception approach to common physical symptoms. Soc Sci Med 2003;57:2343–54.
9. Perlis M, Merica H, Smith M, et al. Beta EEG activity and insomnia. Sleep Med Rev 2001;5:365–76.
10. Jinks JL, Fulker DW. Comparison of the biometrical genetical, MAVA, and classical approaches to the analysis of human behavior. Psychol Bull 1970;73: 311–49.
11. Neale MC, Cardon LR. Methodology for genetic studies of twins and families. Dordrecht (Netherlands): Kluwer Academic Publishers; 1992.
12. Webb WB, Campbell SS. Relationships in sleep characteristics of identical and fraternal twins. Arch Gen Psychiatry 1983;40:1093–5.
13. Partinen M, Kaprio J, Koskenvuo M, et al. Genetic and environmental determination of human sleep. Sleep 1983;6:179–85.
14. Heath A, Kendler K, Eaves L, et al. Evidence for genetic influences on sleep disturbance and sleep pattern in twins. Sleep 1990;13:318–35.
15. Heath A, Eaves L, Kirk K, et al. Effects of lifestyle, personality, symptoms of anxiety and depression, and genetic predisposition on subjective sleep disturbance and sleep pattern. Twin Res 1998;1: 176–88.
16. McCarren M, Goldberg J, Ramakrishnan V, et al. Insomnia in Vietnam era veteran twins: Influence of genes and combat experience. Sleep 1994;17: 456–61.
17. de Castro JM. The influence of heredity on self-reported sleep patterns in free-living humans. Physiol Behav 2002;76:479–86.
18. Watson NF, Goldberg J, Arguelles L, et al. Genetic and environmental influences on insomnia, daytime sleepiness, and obesity in twins. Sleep 2006;29: 645–9.
19. Boomsma DI, van Someren EJ, Beem AL, et al. Sleep during a regular week night: a twin-sibling study. Twin Res Hum Genet 2008;11:538–45.
20. Gregory AM, Eley TC, O'Connor TG, et al. Etiologies of associations between childhood sleep and behavioral problems in a large twin sample. J Am Acad Child Adolesc Psychiatry 2004;43:744–51.
21. Gregory AM, Rijsdijk FV, Eley TC. A twin-study of sleep difficulties in school-aged children. Child Dev 2006;77:1668–79.
22. Gregory AM. A genetic decomposition of the association between parasomnias and dyssomnias in 8-year-old twins. Arch Pediatr Adolesc Med 2008; 162:299–304.
23. Gregory AM, Rijsdijk FV, Dahl RE, et al. Associations between sleep problems, anxiety, and depression in twins at 8 years of age. Pediatrics 2006;118: 1124–32.
24. Gregory AM, Rijsdijk FV, Lau JY, et al. The direction of longitudinal associations between sleep problems and depression symptoms: a study of twins aged 8 and 10 years. Sleep 2009;32:189–99.
25. Abe K, Shimakawa M. Genetic-constitutional factor and childhood insomnia. Psychiatr Neurol (Basel) 1966;152:363–9.
26. Hauri P, Olmstead E. Childhood-onset insomnia. Sleep 1980;3:59–65.
27. Bastien CH, Morin CM. Familial incidence of insomnia. J Sleep Res 2000;9:49–54.
28. Dauvilliers Y, Morin C, Cervena K, et al. Family studies in insomnia. J Psychosom Res 2005;58:271–8.
29. Beaulieu-Bonneau S, LeBlanc M, Merette C, et al. Family history of insomnia in a population-based sample. Sleep 2007;30:1739–45.

30. Drake C, Richardson G, Roehrs T, et al. Vulnerability to stress-related sleep disturbance and hyper-arousal. Sleep 2004;27:285–91.

31. Drake CL, Scofield H, Roth T. Vulnerability to insomnia: the role of familial aggregation. Sleep Med 2008;9:297–302.

32. Lowrey PL, Takahashi JS. Mammalian circadian biology: elucidating genome-wide levels of temporal organization. Annu Rev Genomics Hum Genet 2004; 5:407–41.

33. Laposky A, Easton A, Dugovic C, et al. Deletion of the mammalian circadian clock gene BMAL1/Mop3 alters baseline sleep architecture and the response to sleep deprivation. Sleep 2005;28:395–409.

34. Viola AU, Archer SN, James LM, et al. PER3 polymorphism predicts sleep structure and waking performance. Curr Biol 2007;17:613–8.

35. McClung CA. Circadian genes, rhythms and the biology of mood disorders. Pharmacol Ther 2007; 114:222–32.

36. Serretti A, Benedetti F, Mandelli L, et al. Genetic dissection of psychopathological symptoms: insomnia in mood disorders and CLOCK gene polymorphism. Am J Med Genet B Neuropsychiatr Genet 2003;121: 35–8.

37. Serretti A, Cusin C, Benedetti F, et al. Insomnia improvement during antidepressant treatment and CLOCK gene polymorphism. Am J Med Genet B Neuropsychiatr Genet 2005;137:36–9.

38. Utge SJ, Soronen P, Loukola A, et al. Systematic analysis of circadian genes in a population-based sample reveals association of TIMELESS with depression and sleep disturbance. PLoS One 2010;5:e9259.

39. Perlis RH, Mischoulon D, Smoller JW, et al. Serotonin transporter polymorphisms and adverse effects with fluoxetine treatment. Biol Psychiatry 2003;54:879–83.

40. Brummett BH, Krystal AD, Ashley-Koch A, et al. Sleep quality varies as a function of 5-HTTLPR genotype and stress. Psychosom Med 2007;69: 621–4.

41. Kang RH, Choi MJ, Paik JW, et al. Effect of serotonin receptor 2A gene polymorphism on mirtazapine response in major depression. Int J Psychiatry Med 2007;37:315–29.

42. Brummett BH, Krystal AD, Siegler IC, et al. Associations of a regulatory polymorphism of monoamine oxidase-A gene promoter (MAOA-uVNTR) with symptoms of depression and sleep quality. Psychosom Med 2007;69:396–401.

43. Craig D, Hart DJ, Passmore AP. Genetically increased risk of sleep disruption in Alzheimer's disease. Sleep 2006;29:1003–7.

44. Wisor JP, Nishino S, Sora I, et al. Dopaminergic role in stimulant-induced wakefulness. J Neurosci 2001; 21:1787–94.

45. Kume K, Kume S, Park SK, et al. Dopamine is a regulator of arousal in the fruit fly. J Neurosci 2005;25: 7377–84.

46. Buhr A, Bianchi MT, Baur R, et al. Functional characterization of the new human GABA(A) receptor mutation beta3(R192H). Hum Genet 2002;111: 154–60.

47. Agosto J, Choi JC, Parisky KM, et al. Modulation of GABAA receptor desensitization uncouples sleep onset and maintenance in drosophila. Nat Neurosci 2008;11:354–9.

48. Retey JV, Adam M, Honegger E, et al. A functional genetic variation of adenosine deaminase affects the duration and intensity of deep sleep in humans. Proc Natl Acad Sci U S A 2005;102:15676–81.

49. Retey JV, Adam M, Khatami R, et al. A genetic variation in the adenosine A2A receptor gene (ADORA2A) contributes to individual sensitivity to caffeine effects on sleep. Clin Pharmacol Ther 2007;81:692–8.

50. Gass N, Ollila HM, Utge S, et al. Contribution of adenosine related genes to the risk of depression with disturbed sleep. J Affect Disord 2010;126:134–9.

51. Prober DA, Rihel J, Onah AA, et al. Hypocretin/orexin overexpression induces an insomnia-like phenotype in zebrafish. J Neurosci 2006;26:13400–10.

52. Liu W, Guo F, Lu B, et al. Amnesiac regulates sleep onset and maintenance in Drosophila melanogaster. Biochem Biophys Res Commun 2008; 372:798–803.

53. Gottlieb DJ, O'Connor GT, Wilk JB. Genome-wide association of sleep and circadian phenotypes. BMC Med Genet 2007;8(Suppl 1):S9.

54. Luciano M, Zhu G, Kirk KM, et al. "No thanks, it keeps me awake": the genetics of coffee-attributed sleep disturbance. Sleep 2007;30:1378–86.

55. Wu MN, Koh K, Yue Z, et al. A genetic screen for sleep and circadian mutants reveals mechanisms underlying regulation of sleep in drosophila. Sleep 2008;31:465–72.

56. Seugnet L, Suzuki Y, Thimgan M, et al. Identifying sleep regulatory genes using a drosophila model of insomnia. J Neurosci 2009;29:7148–57.

57. Winrow CJ, Williams DL, Kasarskis A, et al. Uncovering the genetic landscape for multiple sleep-wake traits. PLoS One 2009;4:e5161.

58. McCarthy MI, Hirschhorn JN. Genome-wide association studies: potential next steps on a genetic journey. Hum Mol Genet 2008;17:R156–65.

59. Hindorff LA, Sethupathy P, Junkins HA, et al. Potential etiologic and functional implications of genome-wide association loci for human diseases and traits. Proc Natl Acad Sci U S A 2009;106: 9362–7.

60. Kathiresan S, Willer CJ, Peloso GM, et al. Common variants at 30 loci contribute to polygenic dyslipidemia. Nat Genet 2009;41:56–65.

61. Manolio TA, Collins FS, Cox NJ, et al. Finding the missing heritability of complex diseases. Nature 2009;461:747–53.

62. Maller J, George S, Purcell S, et al. Common variation in three genes, including a noncoding variant in CFH, strongly influences risk of age-related macular degeneration. Nat Genet 2006; 38:1055–9.

63. Zeggini E, Scott LJ, Saxena R, et al. Meta-analysis of genome-wide association data and large-scale replication identifies additional susceptibility loci for type 2 diabetes. Nat Genet 2008;40: 638–45.

64. Benyamin B, McRae AF, Zhu G, et al. Variants in TF and HFE explain approximately 40% of genetic variation in serum-transferrin levels. Am J Hum Genet 2009;84:60–5.

65. Yang J, Benyamin B, McEvoy BP, et al. Common SNPs explain a large proportion of the heritability for human height. Nat Genet 2010;42:565–9.

66. Wray NR. Allele frequencies and the r2 measure of linkage disequilibrium: Impact on design and interpretation of association studies. Twin Res Hum Genet 2005;8:87–94.

67. Falconer D, Mackay T. Introduction to quantitative genetics. Harlow (United Kingdom): Longman; 1996.

Genetics of Restless Legs Syndrome: Mendelian, Complex, and Everything in Between

Barbara Schormair, PhD[a,b], Juliane Winkelmann, MD[a,b,c],*

KEYWORDS

- Restless legs syndrome • Genetics • Complex disease
- Linkage study • Genetic association study

Restless legs syndrome (RLS) is a sleep-related movement disorder with an age-dependent prevalence of up to 10% (ie, one of the most common neurologic illnesses in populations of European descent).[1,2] The defining symptom is an intense and unappeasable urge to move the legs in situations of rest or inactivity, mainly occurring in the evening or at night. Patients usually report unpleasant or even painful sensations deep inside their legs and only moving the extremity leads to an improvement of symptoms. As a consequence, patients with RLS suffer a profound reduction of their overall quality of life because of frequent sleep disruption and subsequent daytime sleepiness.[1,3] They also face an increased occurrence of depression or anxiety and a higher risk of hypertension and cardiovascular disorders.[4,5] Preventive and therapeutic options are necessary for these patients and require detailed knowledge of the underlying molecular processes.

Starting with the first clinical descriptions of RLS by Ekbom[6] in the 1940s, a significant influence of genes on disease susceptibility has been suspected and, over the years, has been proven.[7]

Research followed the classical pathway: simple observation of familial aggregation of the disease; twin studies; and segregation analyses in families to determine the extent of genetic contribution to the phenotype, followed by genome-wide linkage studies in families and, most recently, genome-wide, population-based, case-control association studies to identify the loci involved.

In general, the extent of the genetic predisposition and the number and types of disease-causing variants are different for different diseases. The spectrum extends continuously from mendelian diseases with a single major gene to complex polygenic diseases, where many genes contribute to susceptibility. The underlying risk variants can be classified according to frequency and effect size and range from rare (<1% allele frequency) to common (>5% allele frequency) and from small to large effect size (ie, increasing the risk of disease by a factor of 0.1 or by $\geq$100). Rare variants usually have strong effects, whereas common alleles tend to have small to moderate effect sizes.[8,9]

The view of the genetic architecture of RLS underwent profound changes over the last 20 years.

The authors have nothing to disclose.

[a] Institute of Human Genetics, Helmholtz Zentrum München, German Research Center for Environmental Health, Ingolstaedter Landstrasse 1, Neuherberg 85764, Germany

[b] Institute of Human Genetics, Klinikum Rechts der Isar, Technische Universität München (TUM), Trogerstr. 32, Munich 81675, Germany

[c] Department of Neurology, Klinikum Rechts der Isar, Technische Universität München (TUM), Ismaningerstr, 22, Munich 81675, Germany

* Corresponding author. Klinikum Rechts der Isar, Technische Universität München (TUM), Ismaningerstr, 22, Munich 81675, Germany.

E-mail address: winkelmann@lrz.tu-muenchen.de

Sleep Med Clin 6 (2011) 203–215

doi:10.1016/j.jsmc.2011.04.006

Initially considered to be a mendelian disease with an autosomal-dominant mode of inheritance, it is now perceived as a complex multifactorial disorder, with both genetic and nongenetic factors contributing to the susceptibility. This review is intended to recount this process, thereby summarizing the current status of genetics research in RLS. First cornerstones of the genetic architecture have been uncovered, but the picture is far from complete. In this context, the authors highlight untouched aspects of disease susceptibility mechanisms and discuss the potential of new technologies, such as next-generation sequencing for the genetics of RLS.

THE RLS PHENOTYPE

For any type of genetic analysis, a precise definition of the phenotype under study is required. In the context of disease phenotypes, this means reliable and standardized diagnostic criteria and a comprehensive account of the essential and associated features of the disease. In RLS, the diagnosis is based solely on the patients' description of the clinical symptoms, because there is no objective laboratory test to date. Four essential criteria must be fulfilled for a definite diagnosis of RLS. These criteria represent the key characteristics of the syndrome: (1) the presence of an urge to move the legs, usually accompanied or caused by uncomfortable and unpleasant sensations deep inside the legs; (2) symptoms begin or worsen during rest or inactivity; (3) total or partial relief of symptoms by movement; and (4) symptoms show a diurnal rhythm and are worse in the evening or at night or only occur at this time.[1] In addition to the mandatory criteria, 3 supportive criteria have been devised to further back the diagnosis.[1] The first supportive feature is a positive family history, which is defined as having at least 1 first-degree relative affected with RLS. The second supportive feature is a positive response to dopaminergic treatment because the dopamine precursor levodopa and dopamine-receptor agonists are the first-line therapy option for RLS. The third supportive feature is the presence of periodic limb movements in sleep (PLMS) or while awake, which are present in more than 80% of patients with RLS. Their occurrence, however, is not limited to RLS. Further features generally associated with RLS are a usually progressive course of the disease, the occurrence of sleep disturbances, and a normal physical and neurologic examination.[1]

Besides the idiopathic/primary form of RLS, which accounts for the majority of RLS cases, it is also found as a symptomatic or secondary form concomitant to other medical conditions present in patients.[1,10] The most well-established causes of symptomatic RLS are iron deficiency, pregnancy, and end-stage renal disease. In addition, secondary RLS has been described in Parkinson's disease, type 2 diabetes mellitus, multiple sclerosis, attention-deficit hyperactivity syndrome, and neuropathies.[10–12] Because of overlapping clinical features, shared pathophysiological mechanisms are discussed for both forms.[1] Several candidate pathways and neuroanatomical structures have been suggested, but the exact neuronal cellular processes are still unknown.[13,14] Ever since the discovery of the powerful therapeutic effect of levodopa and dopamine agonists in RLS, the dopaminergic system of the central nervous system (CNS) has been thought to play a role. The involvement of subcortical dopaminergic systems in regulation of motor control and sensory perception further supports this idea because a dysfunction in these pathways could explain both the motor and sensory components of RLS.[14,15] Altered brain iron metabolism has also been proposed as a causal mechanism of RLS.[13,14] Iron deficiency, pregnancy, and end-stage renal disease are the most common causes of symptomatic RLS and all coincide with different derangements in iron status.[11] Treatment with oral or intravenous iron has been shown to ameliorate symptoms.[16] These clinical observations are supported by findings from neuroimaging studies and analyses of iron status and proteins involved in storage and transport of iron in blood and cerebrospinal fluid, which indicate reduced availability of iron in the CNS.[17–19] Neuroimaging and reflex studies suggest a dysfunction in subcortical brain areas leading to reduced supraspinal inhibition and, therefore, increased spinal and, possibly, cortical excitability.[20–22]

Even though standardized diagnostic criteria have been implemented, phenotypic variability remains an issue. Several features of the disease show a broad spectrum. The age of onset of the disorder ranges from early childhood to old age.[23–25] The frequency and severity of symptoms vary from only mild occasional to daily severe symptoms.[1,24] In addition, the course of the disease can be fluctuating with symptom-free episodes or constant with slow progression. Patients can report an emphasis of motor or sensory symptoms.[1,24] From the perspective of genetics, the different manifestations could represent different genetic underpinnings or reflect the influence of nongenetic factors and gene-environment interaction.

To achieve homogeneous patient samples in genetic research, classification schemes are necessary for defining endophenotypes. In RLS, the subtypes established at present have been identified based on the presence (familial RLS) or absence (sporadic RLS) of a positive family history and the age of onset of symptoms (early onset and late-onset RLS).[26] Patients with familial RLS consistently have been shown to have an earlier onset of symptoms compared with sporadic RLS[24,27–30] and, therefore, these criteria can be used in parallel as a marker for the same endophenotype. Three studies have explored the age-of-onset range in patients with RLS and have found a bimodal distribution. The cutoff value between early onset RLS and late-onset RLS was determined either empirically[25,31] or by mathematical modeling[32] and varied between 45, 30, and 36 years. An early age of onset correlates well with a positive family history and idiopathic RLS, whereas a late age of onset is more frequently seen in sporadic and symptomatic RLS.[24,29]

EARLY RLS GENETICS: HERITABILITY AND MODE OF INHERITANCE

Genetics research in RLS was sparked by the observation that a large proportion of patients reported a positive family history. The exact estimates vary from 36.4%[6] up to 92.0%[28] with most studies reporting estimates between 40% and 65%.[23,24,27,32] Familial RLS is also found in symptomatic cases but to a much lower extent than in idiopathic ones (eg, 42.3% vs 11.7%[24]). Such a prominent familial aggregation strongly suggests an underlying genetic basis of the disorder, but the shared environment of the family members alone could also cause the observed aggregation. Systematic approaches, such as pedigree analysis in affected families, twin studies, and complex segregation analyses, followed the early observations of familial aggregation to identify the true genetic contribution and the mode of inheritance of the disease. A common measure of the genetic contribution to a disease is the heritability, which is defined as the fraction of the observed variance of a trait in the population that is explained by genetic factors.[33] Estimates for RLS stem from twin studies and a familial aggregation analysis and range between 54.0% and 69.4%.[34–36] Another measure is the recurrence risk (λ), defined as the risk ratio for a certain type of relative of the affected person compared with the population prevalence.[37] In RLS, one study found a λ of 5.6 for first-degree relatives of patients with RLS.[30] The λ value increased to 6.7 in early onset RLS and decreased to 2.9 in late-onset RLS.[30] Another study looked at specific relative pairs and found a λ of 10.25 for parent-offspring pairs and a λ of 16.23 for siblings.[36] Both measures, therefore, indicate a substantial genetic contribution to RLS.

Early pedigree studies of single families in RLS suggested an autosomal-dominant mode of inheritance with high penetrance and broad variation in expressivity. Age of onset, disease course, frequency and severity of symptoms, and the presence of either both or predominantly sensory or motor symptoms were found to vary considerably within and between families.[38–41] Two of the studies found a decrease in the age of onset in subsequent generations, which was taken as evidence of anticipation in RLS.[40,41] However, as the awareness of the disease is likely to be higher in RLS families, this observation could also simply be an artifact.[7] RLS is also described in patients with spinocerebellar ataxia, a trinucleotide repeat expansion disorder.[42] However, there is no correlation between the length of the repeat and the age of onset, and the data concerning the association of RLS with a pathologic length of the repeat is controversial.[42,43]

Twin studies estimate the extent of the genetic and nongenetic contribution to a trait by comparing the similarity of monozygotic (MZ) and dizygotic (DZ) twins. Three twin studies of varying sample size have been performed in RLS. Ondo and colleagues[44] only looked at MZ twins (n = 12) and found a high concordance rate of 83.3%. Pedigree analysis was in line with the autosomal-dominant mode of inheritance with high penetrance seen in RLS families. However, symptom severity and age of onset showed broad variation within the twin pairs and the sample size was very small.[44] The other studies looked at MZ and DZ twins, and although the exact values for the concordance rates varied, both found higher concordance rates in MZ twins.[34,35] These rates were also less than 100% and, therefore, indicate environmental influences in addition to the genetic ones. Limitations of both studies were recruitment of patients based on self-reported symptoms and use of self-defined diagnostic criteria, which increased the potential for misdiagnosis.[34,35] Nevertheless, all twin studies confirmed the significant genetic contribution to RLS.

Two complex segregation analyses have been performed to systematically investigate the mode of inheritance of RLS. These analyses compare different genetic, nongenetic, and mixed models to the data obtained from family pedigrees and identify the model that fits the data with the highest likelihood. One study in German families (n = 196) recruited only first-degree relatives and stratified patients according to the age of onset of RLS symptoms.[31] The best-fitting model for the early onset group (≤30 years) was an autosomal-dominant model with a single major gene and a significant multifactorial component. For the late-onset group (>30 years) and the whole sample, all but the general model of free transmission probabilities were rejected. The investigators proposed either an oligogenic mode of inheritance with several major genes or substantial environmental influences as the reason for the familial aggregation in their late-onset group.[31] The second study in families (n = 77) from the United States included first- and second-degree relatives and analyzed the whole sample using gender as a covariate.[45] The best-fitting model was an autosomal-dominant model with a single gene and complete penetrance. For the age of onset of RLS, all nongenetic and major gene models were rejected, indicating that age of onset is also controlled by genetic factors and not only by environmental factors.[45] Both studies applied statistical methods to correct for the ascertainment bias that is introduced by recruiting families based on affected family members.

LINKAGE STUDIES: LOOKING FOR MONOGENIC RLS IN FAMILIES

Based on the observations from family, twin, and segregation studies, and the available tools for mapping disease genes at the time, the next step in the genetics' journey in RLS were genome-wide linkage studies. These rely on the detection of a cosegregation of marker loci and the disease in affected families. Marker loci are either microsatellites (mostly short tandem repeats) or single nucleotide polymorphisms (SNPs). Cosegregation occurs because physically close genetic loci are linked and thus inherited together more often than expected by chance. Therefore, markers segregating with the disease in a pedigree indicate the genomic region where the disease-relevant gene or genetic variant is most likely located. The linkage approach is well suited to detect rare variants with strong effects on the phenotype that underlies mendelian diseases. Parametric linkage studies require the specification of a genetic model (mode of inheritance, penetrance, disease allele frequency, phenocopy rate). Nonparametric methods are model free and, thus, more flexible but have less power. The most commonly used statistic for linkage is the logarithm of the odds (LOD) score, where a LOD greater than or equal to 3.3 is necessary to claim statistically significant linkage between marker and disease locus.[46,47]

Both parametric and nonparametric linkage studies have been performed in RLS families from various countries and have identified a total of 6 linkage regions (**Table 1**). The first locus, RLS-1 on chromosome 12q22–23.3, was identified in a genome-wide linkage study of a French Canadian family.[48] Using parametric linkage analysis, a maximum 2-point LOD score of 3.42 and a multipoint LOD score of 3.59 were found. The investigators specified their genetic model as autosomal recessive with a high disease allele frequency of 0.25, a reduced penetrance of 0.8, and a phenocopy rate of 0.005. This model reflects a pseudodominant mode of inheritance, where an increased number of matings between homozygote and heterozygote carriers of the disease allele leads to a seemingly autosomal-dominant pattern in the pedigree. Haplotype and recombination analysis narrowed down the candidate region to 14.71 cM located between markers D12S1044 and D12S78.[43] This finding was confirmed in 5 other French Canadian families with an overall 2-point LOD score of 5.67 and a maximum multipoint LOD score of 8.84, including the first family linked to this locus.[49] They also described an association of the PLMS index to this locus because members of the linked families had significantly increased PLMS indices.[48] Further, weak evidence for linkage to this locus was found in a subset of 12 German families by means of the nonparametric transmission disequilibrium test (TDT) with a P value of .045.[50] Another nonparametric linkage study in the Icelandic population also supports this locus.[51] Here a significant LOD score of 3.88 was reported in subjects with RLS and PLMS or PLMS only, whereas a much smaller LOD score, less than 1, was seen in subjects only positive for the RLS essential criteria.[51]

The second locus, RLS-2 on chromosome 14q13–22, was found in a family originating from Northern Italy.[52] These investigators defined the sole presence of PLMS as an intermediate phenotype of RLS in their analysis. Using an autosomal-dominant mode of inheritance with a disease allele frequency of 0.003, a variable penetrance (0.95 for RLS symptoms, 0.7 for PLMS), and a phenocopy rate of 0.005, they identified a linkage region of 9.1 cM flanked by markers D14S70 and D14S1068. The maximum 2-point LOD score was 3.23 and the maximum nonparametric LOD score was 3.47.[52] A possible confirmation of this locus was presented in a French Canadian family in which suggestive evidence for linkage with LOD scores between 1.46 and 2.51 was found.[53] Interestingly, 2 haplotypes were segregating with the disease, suggesting affected individuals to be compound heterozygotes.[53] A family-based TDT association study of 159 European RLS trios also found significant association to RLS-2 with an empirical P value of .0033.[54]

The third locus, RLS-3 on chromosome 9p24–22, was identified in a study of 15 extended families originating from North America.[36] They delineated

Table 1
Linkage regions for RLS

Locus (OMIM)	Reference	Chromosomal Location	Inheritance Mode	Parametric LOD Score
RLS-1	Desautels et al,[48] 2001	12q22–23.3	AR pseudodominant	3.42 (2P) 3.59 (MP)
RLS-2	Bonati et al,[52] 2003	14q13–22	AD	3.23 (2P)
RLS-3	Chen et al,[36] 2004	9p24–22	AD	3.77 (2P) 3.91 (MP)
RLS-4	Pichler et al,[58] 2006	2q33	AD	4.1 (2P)
RLS-5	Levchenko et al,[59] 2006	20p13	AD	3.34 (2P) 3.86 (MP)
—	Levchenko et al,[61] 2009	16p12.1	AD	3.5 (MP)
—	Winkelmann et al,[62] 2006[a]	4q25–26	AD	2.92 (MP)
—	Winkelmann et al,[62] 2006[a]	17p11–13	AD	2.83 (MP)
—	Kemlink et al,[63] 2008[a]	19p13	AD	2.61 (MP)

The linkage regions for RLS are given with their chromosomal position by chromosome band, the proposed inheritance mode, and the LOD scores from parametric linkage analysis. Both 2-point and multipoint scores are reported. Numbering of loci has been indicated as listed in Online Mendelian Inheritance in Man (OMIM), 1/2010.
 Abbreviations: AD, autosomal dominant; AR, autosomal recessive; MP, multipoint LOD score; 2P, 2-point LOD score.
 [a] Suggestive evidence only.

linkage to this region with a maximum nonparametric linkage score of 3.22. Subsequent parametric linkage analysis based on an autosomal-dominant model with a disease allele frequency of 0.001 and a penetrance of 0.95 confirmed this linkage signal in 2 families. The maximum 2-point and multipoint LOD scores of the combined analysis of these 2 families were 3.77 and 3.91, respectively. Haplotype and recombination analysis defined the critical region between markers D9S1779 and D9S162.[36] The statistical methodology of this study and, thus, the significance of the linkage result have been questioned,[55] but several subsequent studies have confirmed the RLS-3 region. Parametric linkage analysis in a German family based on the parameters from the segregation analysis in German families[31] revealed a maximum 2-point LOD score of 3.88 and maximum multipoint LOD score of 3.78.[56] The critical region could be reduced to 11.1 cM between markers D9S256 and D9S157. The investigators assumed intrafamilial heterogeneity and stratified their sample based on the age of onset. Only early onset RLS cases (≤32 years) were classified as affected in the analysis.[56] Marginally significant association to RLS-3 was found in South European and Central European RLS trios by means of a TDT.[54] Further evidence for an RLS locus on chromosome 9 originates from a parametric linkage analysis of an extended German family.[57] Using an autosomal-dominant model with a disease allele frequency of 0.003,

complete penetrance, and a phenocopy rate of 0.005, the investigators found a maximum multipoint LOD score of 3.6 for a 20 cM region centromeric of the original RLS-3 locus and termed this region RLS-3*.[57] The LOD score for the original RLS-3 locus was 1.3, indicating that linkage to this region could not be excluded in this family. Haplotype analysis showed a haplotype comprising the new region and the centromeric part of the original RLS-3 signal, which was shared by all but 1 family member. The phenotype of this individual is unclear and, accordingly, the existence of a truly new linkage locus centromeric to RLS-3 could be questioned. However, the haplotype shared by all unequivocally affected family members confirms the centromeric part of RLS-3.[57]

The fourth locus, RLS-4 on chromosome 2q33, was identified in 3 families of an isolated population in South Tyrol in Italy.[58] Parametric linkage analysis was based on an autosomal-dominant mode of inheritance, a disease allele frequency of 0.001, a penetrance of 0.7, and a phenocopy rate of 0.01, and allowed for locus heterogeneity. A maximum parametric 2-point LOD score of 5.1 was found, and the nonparametric analysis disclosed a maximum LOD score of 5.5. The initial candidate region of 11.7 cM was narrowed to 8.2 cM between markers D2S311 and D2S2208 by haplotype and recombination analysis.[58]

The fifth locus, RLS-5 on chromosome 20p13, was revealed in a French Canadian family.[59] The genetic model for the parametric linkage analysis included an autosomal-dominant mode of inheritance, a disease allele frequency of 0.001, a penetrance of 0.7, and a phenocopy rate of 0.001. Two-point and multipoint analysis yielded maximum LOD scores of 3.34 and 3.86. The critical region spans 16 cM and is flanked by the telomeric end of chromosome 20 and marker D20S835.[59] It was confirmed in a Dutch kindred in a parametric linkage analysis applying a model of autosomal-dominant inheritance, a disease allele frequency of 0.005, a penetrance of 0.99, and a phenocopy rate of 0.01.[60] The investigators stratified affection status according to symptom severity and included only severely affected individuals. A peak multipoint LOD score of 3.02 was found at marker D20S116 in the RLS-5 region with the critical region of 13 cM (4.5 Mb) flanked by the markers CGR490 and rs2065704.[60]

An additional, not-yet-named linkage locus was found on chromosome 16p12.1, also in a French Canadian family.[61] Again, parametric linkage analysis was performed and yielded a maximum multipoint LOD score of 3.5 for a candidate region of 1.18 Mb split into 2 parts by a double recombination. Suggestive evidence for this locus was found in a smaller French Canadian family in the same study.[61]

Suggestive evidence of linkage exists for 3 other loci. Two were identified in a single large German family using an autosomal-dominant model in a parametric linkage analysis.[62] One locus is located on chromosome 4q25–26 with a maximum multipoint LOD score of 2.92. The other locus on 17p11–13 showed a maximum multipoint LOD score of 2.83. The latter locus was corroborated by evidence of linkage found in European RLS trios.[62] A third locus was shown on chromosome 19p13 in an Italian family with a maximum parametric LOD score of 2.61, assuming an autosomal-dominant mode of inheritance.[63]

Although these studies establish that mendelian forms of RLS, mostly with an autosomal-dominant mode of inheritance, exist, the underlying genetic model is not simple. There is substantial locus heterogeneity and considerable interfamilial and intrafamilial variation in the clinical presentation of symptoms.[41,49,56] The LOD scores found are lower than what would be expected in these pedigrees based on simulations.[7,56] Moreover, families have been described where more than 50% of the offspring are affected, and in other families no linkage could be found.[49,50] In summary, this points to a complex system consisting of major loci and additional smaller effect and modifier genes.

The identified linkage regions are quite large, encompassing several megabases of sequence, and, hence, also a large number of genes (eg,

more than 300 in the RLS-1 region). Therefore, only a few candidate genes were sequenced in the linked families to look for causal mutations (**Table 2**). The selection of genes was driven by the supposed pathophysiology and includes CNS ion channels, neuronal transcription factors, and genes involved in iron and dopamine metabolism. For none of these genes, causal mutations segregating with the disease in the families under study were found. However, sequencing was limited mainly to exons and splice sites and noncoding elements, such as introns, and 5' and 3' untranslated regions were not sequenced in most genes.

ASSOCIATION STUDIES: IT IS GETTING COMPLEX

Association studies are tailored to a different type of susceptibility variants than linkage studies. They are powerful tools for detecting common variants with moderate to small effects on disease risk, which are thought to underlie common complex diseases (the so-called common disease, common variant hypothesis).[64] Here, allele or genotype frequencies of genetic variants, usually SNPs, are compared between affected (cases) and unaffected subjects (controls). A variant is associated with a disease if there is a statistically significant difference in the frequencies between affected and unaffected individuals.[65] These studies used to be limited to individual candidate genes and only in the past 5 years have become feasible on a genome-wide level because of technological and methodological advances.[64] Large-scale studies are enabled by the existence of linkage disequilibrium (LD) between SNPs. Being in LD means that the genotypes of 2 or more SNPs correlate tightly and one can serve as a proxy (tagging SNP) for the other, thereby reducing the total number of SNPs that have to be tested.[65,66] For valid results, these studies must take into account problems, such as false-positive associations caused by the simultaneous testing of multiple hypotheses or caused by population stratification. In addition, associations should be confirmed in independent case-control populations (replication).[65,66]

Candidate-Gene Association Studies

The variants tested in candidate-gene studies were selected either as pathophysiological candidates potentially involved in RLS in accordance with the disease hypothesis or as physical candidates located in one of the previously identified linkage regions. The first candidate-gene study investigated genes involved in dopaminergic transmission and dopamine metabolism: the dopamine receptors (*DRD1-5*), the dopamine

Table 2
Candidate genes investigated in RLS linkage regions

Gene	Linkage Region	Method	Reference
NTS	RLS-1	Sequencing of exons and splice sites in 9 affected and 10 unaffected subjects from 4 unrelated families	Desautels et al,[91] 2004
DMT1	RLS-1[a]	Sequencing of exons and regulatory sequences in 4 affected subjects	Xiong et al,[68] 2007
MUPP1 SLC1A1 KCNV2	RLS-3	Sequencing of exons and splice sites, number of sequenced subjects not given	Chen et al,[36] 2004
ELAVL2 CDKN2B TEK	RLS-3*	Sequencing of exons and splice sites in 2 affected family members	Lohmann-Hedrich et al,[57] 2008
SDCBP2 SNPH ProSAPiP1 NRSN2 PDYN ZCCH3 TCF15 SCRT2 ZNF343 PANK2 SRXN1 PTPRA	RLS-5	Sequencing of exons, splice sites, and 5' and 3' untranslated regions in 2 affected and 1 unaffected family members	Sas et al,[60] 2010
HS3ST2 USP31 SCNN1G SCNN1B COG7 GGA2 AQP8 ZKSCAN2	16p12.1	Sequencing of exons, splice sites, and promoter regions in 2 affected family members	Levchenko et al,[61] 2009
KCNN1 RAB3A	19p13	Sequencing of exons and splice sites in 3 affected family members	Kemlink et al,[63] 2008

[a] This gene is not included in the original RLS-1 region, but according to Xiong and colleagues,[68] the study by Hicks and colleagues[51] indicated different limits of this region, which then also included DMT1.

transporter (DAT), and the enzymes tyrosine hydroxylase (TH) and dopamine β-hydroxylase (DBH).[67] Eight known functional polymorphisms in these genes were analyzed in 92 RLS cases and 182 controls from the French Canadian population, but no significant association was found. Stratification of the cases based on age of onset or the PLMS index did not alter the results.[67]

A total of 10 SNPs distributed throughout the divalent metal transporter DMT1, important in cellular iron absorption and located in close proximity to the RLS-1 linkage region, were analyzed in 179 cases and 180 controls, also of French Canadian ancestry. No association to RLS was found.[68]

Most recently, a known functional polymorphism in the catechol-O-methyltransferase gene, which is involved in the degradation of catecholamines, such as dopamine, was genotyped in 298 cases and 135 controls from Germany and showed no significant association.[69]

However, none of these genes can definitely be excluded as candidate genes in RLS because they contain many other potentially etiologic variants not yet assessed.

The only positive candidate-gene study so far targeted the monoamine oxidase isoenzymes MAOA and MAOB, which degrade dopamine and other neuroactive amines.[70] A functional variable number of tandem repeats polymorphism in the MAOA and a dinucleotide repeat in the MAOB gene were genotyped in 96 French Canadian RLS cases and 200 controls. The investigators found an association of the high transcription activity MAOA allele to RLS only in women (odds ratio

[OR] = 2, 95% confidence interval [CI] = 1.06–3.77).[70] This result still awaits confirmation in an independent case-control population.

Association Studies in RLS Linkage Regions

To date, 2 of the known linkage regions, RLS-1 on chromosome 12 and RLS-3 on chromosome 9, have been screened in population-based case-control association studies.[71,72]

The RLS-1 study was conducted in a 3-stage design using cases and controls of European descent recruited in Germany.[71] In an explorative phase, 1536 tagging SNPs and nonsynonymous and synonymous coding and splice-site SNPs in 366 genes contained in the RLS1 region were genotyped in 367 cases and 367 controls. The most significantly associated 24 SNPs from this stage were genotyped in an independent case-control sample (551 cases/551 controls) in the replication phase. SNP rs7977109 in the NOS1 (nNOS) gene was significantly associated with the RLS phenotype (P value = .049, OR = 0.76 with 95% CI = 0.64–0.9). Subsequent high-density analysis of this gene left 3 SNPs in the explorative sample (rs4766836, rs2293054, rs6490121) and 3 SNPs in the replication sample (rs7977109, rs530393, rs816292) as significantly associated after correction for multiple testing.[71] The interpretation of these results is not straightforward because different SNPs located in different parts of the gene are associated in the 2 samples. Further studies are needed to clarify this issue, but this is the first evidence for an association of variants in NOS1 with RLS. From the point of view of gene function, NOS1 is an interesting candidate for RLS. It catalyzes the synthesis of nitric oxide and its action in the CNS has been associated with pain perception, the control of sleep wake regulation, and the modulation of dopaminergic transmission.[73,74]

For the RLS-3 study, a target region of 31 Mb on the short arm of chromosome 9 (9p, 0.5–31.5 Mb), encompassing all published linkage peaks for RLS-3, was defined and a 2-stage case-control association study was performed.[72] In the explorative stage, 628 cases and 1644 controls recruited in Germany were genotyped on commodity SNP arrays with 3270 SNPs located in the RLS-3 region. Eight SNPs were chosen for replication in the second stage and genotyped in independent German (1271 cases/1901 controls), Czech (279/368), and Canadian (285/842) samples. Two SNPs, rs1975197 and rs4626664, were associated with RLS after correction for multiple testing (rs4626664: P value = .00012, OR = 1.44; rs1975197: P value = .0012, OR = 1.31).[72] The

SNPs are located 0.41 Mb apart and map to introns of the gene protein tyrosine phosphatase receptor type delta (PTPRD). They represent 2 independent association signals and, therefore, 2 independent risk variants for RLS within the same locus.[72] Studies in PTPRD knockout mice showed a function of this protein in long-term potentiation in memory formation and in axon guidance and termination of mammalian motorneurons during embryonic development.[75,76] The involvement and function in RLS is still unknown.

It should be noted that the identified associations on chromosome 12q and 9p cannot account for the previously identified linkage signals in the same regions because their effect size is too small to be responsible for a mendelian segregation pattern in families. In both studies, exons and splice sites of the respective genes NOS1 and PTPRD were sequenced in individuals from linked families to identify the underlying causal variant. However, no such variant segregating with disease was found.[71,72]

Genome-wide Association Studies

Two simultaneously published genome-wide association studies (GWAS) have been performed for RLS, one in German and French Canadian cases and the other in cases from Iceland and the United States.[77,78]

The German study analyzed a total of 236,758 SNPs genome-wide in 401 cases and 1644 population-based controls.[77] Variants distributed over 6 genomic loci were carried forward to the replication stage and genotyped in 2 independent samples, a further German (903 cases/891 controls) and a French Canadian sample (255/287). Three loci were significantly associated with RLS after correction for multiple testing: 2 intronic SNPs in MEIS1 on chromosome 2p (P value = 8.1×10^{-23}, OR = 1.74), 5 intronic SNPs in BTBD9 on chromosome 6p (P value = 9.4×10^{-13}, OR = 1.67), and 7 intronic or intergenic SNPs in a region on chromosome 15q containing the 3' end of the MAP2K5 gene and the adjacent SKOR1 (formerly named LBXCOR1) gene (P value = 2.5×10^{-10}, OR = 1.51). A specific combination of risk alleles (haplotype) in MEIS1 was found to have a larger effect than the individual SNPs (OR = 2.7), suggesting the existence of more than 1 risk variant at this locus.[77] The associated genes MEIS1, BTBD9, and MAP2K5/SKOR1 had never been considered as candidates based on previous biologic knowledge. Regarding BTBD9, knowledge of gene function is limited, whereas the other genes have been described in developmental processes, such as limb axis formation (MEIS1),[79] neuronal differentiation (MEIS1, SKOR1),[80,81] and muscle cell differentiation (MAP2K5).[82]

The association to BTBD9 was also reported in the Icelandic GWAS.[78] A total of 306 cases and 15,664 controls from Iceland were analyzed for 306,937 SNPs, followed by a replication in a second Icelandic sample (123 cases/1233 controls) and a US sample (188/662). Only SNPs in the BTBD9 gene were significantly associated (rs3923809, $P = 3 \times 10^{-14}$, OR = 1.7). The phenotypic characterization of cases included the ascertainment of the presence of PLMS, enabling the authors to stratify their sample into RLS cases with and without PLMS. The association of rs3923809 was only found in RLS with PLMS, suggesting an involvement of this locus in the development of PLMS. In addition, this SNP was associated with serum ferritin levels in RLS patients with a decrease of 13% per copy of the risk allele ($P = .002$), suggesting a function in iron storage.[78] The involvement of BTBD9 in iron metabolism might be limited to the RLS phenotype because this gene has not been identified as a genetic factor determining iron metabolism,[83] and replication is also pending.

The differing results from both GWAS might be explained by the respective case ascertainment strategies. In the German study, all patients were diagnosed in a face-to-face interview by expert clinicians, whereas the Icelandic study used a self-administered questionnaire incorporating the essential diagnostic criteria.[77,78] Reassessment of status in face-to-face interviews in a subset revealed a false-positive rate of 22.7%.[78]

The associations found in the GWAS have been substantiated by independent follow-up investigations. The association of MEIS1 and BTBD9 was confirmed in a case-control sample (244/497) from the United States[84] and that of all 3 loci in a mixed sample of European descent including Czech, Austrian, and Finnish cases and controls (1298/2460).[85]

THE GENETICS OF RLS: CURRENT STATUS AND NEXT STEPS

Two main aspects should be considered when trying to evaluate the current status of RLS genetics. One is progress related to our understanding of the genetic architecture of the disease (ie, the number and type of risk variants that exist). The other is the translation of genetic findings into functional knowledge and into a benefit for the patients such as via new therapeutics or risk prediction and the development of appropriate preventive measures.

Substantial progress has been made regarding the idea of the genetic model of RLS. Linkage studies have established mendelian forms of RLS,

mostly with a major genetic factor segregating in an autosomal-dominant fashion. However, it was also recognized that in addition to a major gene, other genetic and nongenetic factors play a modifying role in these forms. The observed locus heterogeneity, the variable penetrance and expressivity, and the phenotypic diversity support this notion. Mendelian-type RLS does not account for the high prevalence of the disease. In the majority of cases, the genetic basis is assumed to be that of a common complex genetic disease, where many common variants with small effect size contribute to disease susceptibility (CDCV hypothesis).[86] Owing to the advent of large-scale, SNP-based, case-control association studies, several such variants have been identified for RLS. These variants have a risk allele frequency of 10% to 30% and mostly small effect sizes, increasing the risk for disease by 0.3 to 0.7 (ie, 1 risk allele will increase your risk of RLS from 10% to 17%).[77,78]

The functional translation is progressing more slowly. One obvious obstruction is the fact that the causally related genes and the etiologic variants in these genes are largely still elusive. Within linkage regions, no causal gene has been identified as of yet, and the associated variants found by GWAS or focused association studies are most likely not the etiologic variants but merely markers correlated with them because of LD. Association studies have at least narrowed down individual genes that are likely causally related. Nevertheless, there is the remote possibility that the association signals are within long-range regulatory elements belonging to more distant genes. First functional studies of the identified genes and the associated variants have been conducted, but do not allow definite conclusions. A study in French Canadian patients with RLS indicated that the MEIS1 risk haplotype influences RNA and protein levels of MEIS1 supporting a functional role of the SNP or the region tagged by the haplotype and of MEIS1 in RLS etiology.[87] Some of the identified RLS genes, such as MEIS1, are known to be involved in embryonic development of the CNS and determination of cell fate at early embryonic stages.[81,88] The role and time point of involvement in RLS is unknown. The only other hint at a function of an associated variant is the correlation of rs3923809 within BTBD9 with serum ferritin levels observed in the Icelandic GWAS,[78] but, apparently, this is not an affect that can be generalized to iron metabolism on the whole.[83] The functional characterization aims at a better understanding of the molecular mechanism leading to the disease, and, in the future, at developing new therapeutic approaches. Another area of application of genetic data is risk prediction, which, optimally, would enable preventive measures. For RLS, such predictions can only be based on the associated variants. Today, because of their small effects, their relevance for risk prediction at an individual level is limited. This finding was shown by an area under the receiver operating characteristic curve analysis, where the classification based on number of risk alleles in 4 RLS-associated genes (*MEIS1*, *BTBD9*, *MAP2K5/SKOR1*, and *PTPRD*) was not significantly better than random assignment of disease status.[72]

What could be the next steps in the study of genetics of RLS? The loci identified so far only partly explain the genetic contribution to RLS, and additional risk variants remain to be discovered. The rare variants with strong effects underlying the linkage regions are specific to the individual family. The common variants found by association studies can explain a large proportion of the risk in the general population because of their high frequency, as evidenced by a population attributable risk fraction of 68.6% for the variants identified in *MEIS1*, *BTBD9*, and *MAP2K5/SKOR1* in the German population.[77] However, these variants only account for a minute fraction of the familial aggregation and heritability of RLS (~3%, Winkelmann and colleagues, unpublished data, 2011), which is a common observation in complex disease genetics.[89] Several potential sources of risk variants exist and could sum up to explain this missing heritability.[89] On the one hand, further common risk variants are expected to be found with GWAS of increasing sample size and number of SNP markers, and RLS is obviously a phenotype well suited to this type of study. On the other hand, certain types of genetic variation have not yet been studied in RLS such as structural variation (eg, copy number variants) or epigenetic modifications (eg, methylation and histone acetylation). Gene-gene interaction and gene-environment interaction are further possible, not-yet-assessed contributors. Symptomatic RLS could be a fitting model system for gene-environment interactions because it is strongly dependent on environmental triggers. Apart from genetics, we should keep in mind that the environmental factors still have to be discovered.

A promising new technology for RLS genetics research is next-generation sequencing, where massive parallel sequencing generates huge amounts of data within a short time and at a comparatively low cost.[90] Within the next years, sequencing of large genomic regions, such as the linkage regions, all known coding regions (the exome), or even the whole genome, will become routine practice. This method will allow the detection of the whole spectrum of genetic variation,

such as rare variants not accessible to the GWAS approach and variants of too small effect size to give rise to a linkage peak. It will take time to develop the necessary analytical tools and cheap high-throughput techniques, but this future is not too far away.

REFERENCES

1. Allen RP, Picchietti D, Hening WA, et al. Restless legs syndrome: diagnostic criteria, special considerations, and epidemiology. A report from the restless legs syndrome diagnosis and epidemiology workshop at the National Institutes of Health. Sleep Med 2003;4:101–19.
2. Berger K, Kurth T. RLS epidemiology–frequencies, risk factors and methods in population studies. Mov Disord 2007;22:S420–3.
3. Hening WA, Allen RP, Chaudhuri KR, et al. Clinical significance of RLS. Mov Disord 2007;22:S395–400.
4. Winkelman JW, Shahar E, Sharief I, et al. Association of restless legs syndrome and cardiovascular disease in the Sleep Heart Health Study. Neurology 2008;70:35–42.
5. Walters AS, Rye DB. Review of the relationship of restless legs syndrome and periodic limb movements in sleep to hypertension, heart disease, and stroke. Sleep 2009;32:589–97.
6. Ekbom K. Restless legs: a clinical study. Acta Med Scand Suppl 1945;158:1–123.
7. Winkelmann J, Polo O, Provini F, et al. Genetics of restless legs syndrome (RLS): state-of-the-art and future directions. Mov Disord 2007;22:S449–58.
8. Botstein D, Risch N. Discovering genotypes underlying human phenotypes: past successes for mendelian disease, future approaches for complex disease. Nat Genet 2003;(Suppl 33):228–37.
9. Schork NJ, Murray SS, Frazer KA, et al. Common vs. rare allele hypotheses for complex diseases. Curr Opin Genet Dev 2009;19:212–9.
10. Merlino G, Valente M, Serafini A, et al. Restless legs syndrome: diagnosis, epidemiology, classification and consequences. Neurol Sci 2007;28:S37–46.
11. Garcia-Borreguero D, Egatz R, Winkelmann J, et al. Epidemiology of restless legs syndrome: the current status. Sleep Med Rev 2006;10:153–67.
12. Cortese S, Konofal E, Lecendreux M, et al. Restless legs syndrome and attention-deficit/hyperactivity disorder: a review of the literature. Sleep 2005;28:1007–13.
13. Paulus W, Dowling P, Rijsman R, et al. Update of the pathophysiology of the restless-legs-syndrome. Mov Disord 2007;22:S431–9.
14. Winkelman JW. Considering the causes of RLS. Eur J Neurol 2006;13(Suppl 3):8–14.
15. Paulus W, Dowling P, Rijsman R, et al. Pathophysiological concepts of restless legs syndrome. Mov Disord 2007;22:1451–6.

16. Allen RP, Earley CJ. The role of iron in restless legs syndrome. Mov Disord 2007;22:S440–8.

17. Mizuno S, Mihara T, Miyaoka T, et al. CSF iron, ferritin and transferrin levels in restless legs syndrome. J Sleep Res 2005;14:43–7.

18. Earley CJ, B Barker P, Horská A, et al. MRI-determined regional brain iron concentrations in early- and late-onset restless legs syndrome. Sleep Med 2006;7:458–61.

19. Allen RP, Barker PB, Wehrl F, et al. MRI measurement of brain iron in patients with restless legs syndrome. Neurology 2001;56:263–5.

20. Bara-Jimenez W, Aksu M, Graham B, et al. Periodic limb movements in sleep: state-dependent excitability of the spinal flexor reflex. Neurology 2000;54:1609–16.

21. Scalise A, Cadore IP, Gigli GL. Motor cortex excitability in restless legs syndrome. Sleep Med 2004;5:393–6.

22. Stiasny-Kolster K, Haeske H, Tergau F, et al. Cortical silent period is shortened in restless legs syndrome independently from circadian rhythm. Suppl Clin Neurophysiol 2003;56:381–9.

23. Walters AS, Hickey K, Maltzman J, et al. A questionnaire study of 138 patients with restless legs syndrome: the 'Night-Walkers' survey. Neurology 1996;46:92–5.

24. Winkelmann J, Wetter TC, Collado-Seidel V, et al. Clinical characteristics and frequency of the hereditary restless legs syndrome in a population of 300 patients. Sleep 2000;23:597–602.

25. Allen RP, Earley CJ. Defining the phenotype of the restless legs syndrome (RLS) using age-of-symptom-onset. Sleep Med 2000;1:11–9.

26. Allen RP, Earley CJ. Restless legs syndrome: a review of clinical and pathophysiologic features. J Clin Neurophysiol 2001;18:128–47.

27. Montplaisir J, Boucher S, Poirier G, et al. Clinical, polysomnographic, and genetic characteristics of restless legs syndrome: a study of 133 patients diagnosed with new standard criteria. Mov Disord 1997;12:61–5.

28. Ondo W, Jankovic J. Restless legs syndrome: clinicoetiologic correlates. Neurology 1996;47:1435–41.

29. Hanson M, Honour M, Singleton A, et al. Analysis of familial and sporadic restless legs syndrome in age of onset, gender, and severity features. J Neurol 2004;251:1398–401.

30. Allen RP, La Buda MC, Becker P, et al. Family history study of the restless legs syndrome. Sleep Med 2002;(Suppl 3):S3–7.

31. Winkelmann J, Muller-Myhsok B, Wittchen HU, et al. Complex segregation analysis of restless legs syndrome provides evidence for an autosomal dominant mode of inheritance in early age at onset families. Ann Neurol 2002;52:297–302.

32. Whittom S, Dauvilliers Y, Pennestri MH, et al. Age-at-onset in restless legs syndrome: a clinical and polysomnographic study. Sleep Med 2007;9:54–9.

33. Visscher PM, Hill WG, Wray NR. Heritability in the genomics era–concepts and misconceptions. Nat Rev Genet 2008;9:255–66.

34. Desai AV, Cherkas LF, Spector TD, et al. Genetic influences in self-reported symptoms of obstructive sleep apnoea and restless legs: a twin study. Twin Res 2004;7:589–95.

35. Xiong L, Jang K, Montplaisir J, et al. Canadian restless legs syndrome twin study. Neurology 2007;68:1631–3.

36. Chen S, Ondo WG, Rao S, et al. Genome-wide linkage scan identifies a novel susceptibility locus for restless legs syndrome on chromosome 9p. Am J Hum Genet 2004;74:876–85.

37. Risch N. Linkage strategies for genetically complex traits. I. Multilocus models. Am J Hum Genet 1990;46:222–8.

38. Walters AS, Picchietti D, Hening W, et al. Variable expressivity in familial restless legs syndrome. Arch Neurol 1990;47:1219–20.

39. Montplaisir J, Godbout R, Boghen D, et al. Familial restless legs with periodic movements in sleep: electrophysiologic, biochemical, and pharmacologic study. Neurology 1985;35:130–4.

40. Trenkwalder C, Seidel VC, Gasser T, et al. Clinical symptoms and possible anticipation in a large kindred of familial restless legs syndrome. Mov Disord 1996;11:389–94.

41. Lazzarini A, Walters AS, Hickey K, et al. Studies of penetrance and anticipation in five autosomal-dominant restless legs syndrome pedigrees. Mov Disord 1999;14:111–6.

42. Konieczny M, Bauer P, Tomiuk J, et al. CAG repeats in restless legs syndrome. Am J Med Genet B Neuropsychiatr Genet 2006;141B:173–6.

43. Desautels A, Turecki G, Montplaisir J, et al. Analysis of CAG repeat expansions in restless legs syndrome. Sleep 2003;26:1055–7.

44. Ondo WG, Vuong KD, Wang Q. Restless legs syndrome in monozygotic twins: clinical correlates. Neurology 2000;55:1404–6.

45. Mathias RA, Hening W, Washburn M, et al. Segregation analysis of restless legs syndrome: possible evidence for a major gene in a family study using blinded diagnoses. Hum Hered 2006;62:157–64.

46. Lander ES, Kruglyak L. Genetic dissection of complex traits: guidelines for interpreting and reporting linkage results. Nat Genet 1995;11(3):241–7.

47. Dawn Teare M, Barrett JH. Genetic linkage studies. Lancet 2005;366(9490):1036–44.

48. Desautels A, Turecki G, Montplaisir J, et al. Identification of a major susceptibility locus for restless legs syndrome on chromosome 12q. Am J Hum Genet 2001;69:1266–70.

49. Desautels A, Turecki G, Montplaisir J, et al. Restless legs syndrome: confirmation of linkage to

chromosome 12q, genetic heterogeneity, and evidence of complexity. Arch Neurol 2005;62:591–6.

50. Winkelmann J, Lichtner P, Putz B, et al. Evidence for further genetic locus heterogeneity and confirmation of RLS-1 in restless legs syndrome. Mov Disord 2006;21:28–33.

51. Hicks A, Rye D, Kristjansson K, et al. Population-based confirmation of the 12q RLS locus in Iceland. Mov Disord 2005;20:S34.

52. Bonati MT, Ferini-Strambi L, Aridon P, et al. Autosomal dominant restless legs syndrome maps on chromosome 14q. Brain 2003;126:1485–92.

53. Levchenko A, Montplaisir JY, Dube MP, et al. The 14q restless legs syndrome locus in the French Canadian population. Ann Neurol 2004;55:887–91.

54. Kemlink D, Polo O, Montagna P, et al. Family-based association study of the restless legs syndrome loci 2 and 3 in a European population. Mov Disord 2007; 22:207–12.

55. Ray A, Weeks DE. No convincing evidence of linkage for restless legs syndrome on chromosome 9p. Am J Hum Genet 2005;76:705–7 [author reply: 707–10].

56. Liebetanz KM, Winkelmann J, Trenkwalder C, et al. RLS3: fine-mapping of an autosomal dominant locus in a family with intrafamilial heterogeneity. Neurology 2006;67:320–1.

57. Lohmann-Hedrich K, Neumann A, Kleensang A, et al. Evidence for linkage of restless legs syndrome to chromosome 9p: are there two distinct loci? Neurology 2008;70:686–94.

58. Pichler I, Marroni F, Volpato CB, et al. Linkage analysis identifies a novel locus for restless legs syndrome on chromosome 2q in a South Tyrolean population isolate. Am J Hum Genet 2006;79: 716–23.

59. Levchenko A, Provost S, Montplaisir JY, et al. A novel autosomal dominant restless legs syndrome locus maps to chromosome 20p13. Neurology 2006; 67:900–1.

60. Sas AM, Di Fonzo A, Bakker SL, et al. Autosomal dominant restless legs syndrome maps to chromosome 20p13 (RLS-5) in a Dutch kindred. Mov Disord 2010;25:1715–22.

61. Levchenko A, Montplaisir JY, Asselin G, et al. Autosomal-dominant locus for restless legs syndrome in French-Canadians on chromosome 16p12.1. Mov Disord 2009;24:40–50.

62. Winkelmann J, Lichtner P, Kemlink D, et al. New loci for restless legs syndrome map to chromosome 4q and 17p. Mov Disord 2006;21:S412.

63. Kemlink D, Plazzi G, Vetrugno R, et al. Suggestive evidence for linkage for restless legs syndrome on chromosome 19p13. Neurogenetics 2008;9:75–82.

64. Altshuler D, Daly MJ, Lander ES. Genetic mapping in human disease. Science 2008;322:881–8.

65. Hirschhorn JN, Daly MJ. Genome-wide association studies for common diseases and complex traits. Nat Rev Genet 2005;6:95–108.

66. McCarthy MI, Abecasis GR, Cardon LR, et al. Genome-wide association studies for complex traits: consensus, uncertainty and challenges. Nat Rev Genet 2008;9:356–69.

67. Desautels A, Turecki G, Montplaisir J, et al. Dopaminergic neurotransmission and restless legs syndrome: a genetic association analysis. Neurology 2001;57:1304–6.

68. Xiong L, Dion P, Montplaisir J, et al. Molecular genetic studies of DMT1 on 12q in French-Canadian restless legs syndrome patients and families. Am J Med Genet B Neuropsychiatr Genet 2007; 144B:911–7.

69. Mylius V, Moller JC, Strauch K, et al. No significance of the COMT val158met polymorphism in restless legs syndrome. Neurosci Lett 2010;473:151–4.

70. Desautels A, Turecki G, Montplaisir J, et al. Evidence for a genetic association between monoamine oxidase A and restless legs syndrome. Neurology 2002;59:215–9.

71. Winkelmann J, Lichtner P, Schormair B, et al. Variants in the neuronal nitric oxide synthase (nNOS, NOS1) gene are associated with restless legs syndrome. Mov Disord 2008;23:350–8.

72. Schormair B, Kemlink D, Roeske D, et al. PTPRD (protein tyrosine phosphatase receptor type delta) is associated with restless legs syndrome. Nat Genet 2008;40:946–8.

73. Gautier-Sauvigne S, Colas D, Parmantier P, et al. Nitric oxide and sleep. Sleep Med Rev 2005;9:101–13.

74. West AR, Galloway MP, Grace AA. Regulation of striatal dopamine neurotransmission by nitric oxide: effector pathways and signaling mechanisms. Synapse 2002;44:227–45.

75. Uetani N, Chagnon MJ, Kennedy TE, et al. Mammalian motoneuron axon targeting requires receptor protein tyrosine phosphatases sigma and delta. J Neurosci 2006;26:5872–80.

76. Uetani N, Kato K, Ogura H, et al. Impaired learning with enhanced hippocampal long-term potentiation in PTPdelta-deficient mice. EMBO J 2000;19:2775–85.

77. Winkelmann J, Schormair B, Lichtner P, et al. Genome-wide association study of restless legs syndrome identifies common variants in three genomic regions. Nat Genet 2007;39:1000–6.

78. Stefansson H, Rye DB, Hicks A, et al. A genetic risk factor for periodic limb movements in sleep. N Engl J Med 2007;357:639–47.

79. Mercader N, Leonardo E, Azpiazu N, et al. Conserved regulation of proximodistal limb axis development by Meis1/Hth. Nature 1999;402:425–9.

80. Mizuhara E, Nakatani T, Minaki Y, et al. Corl1, a novel neuronal lineage-specific transcriptional corepressor for the homeodomain transcription factor Lbx1. J Biol Chem 2005;280:3645–55.

81. Maeda R, Mood K, Jones TL, et al. Xmeis1, a proto-oncogene involved in specifying neural crest cell fate in Xenopus embryos. Oncogene 2001;20: 1329–42.

82. Dinev D, Jordan BW, Neufeld B, et al. Extracellular signal regulated kinase 5 (ERK5) is required for the differentiation of muscle cells. EMBO Rep 2001;2:829–34.

83. Oexle K, Ried JS, Hicks AA, et al. Novel association to the proprotein convertase PCSK7 gene locus revealed by analysing soluble transferrin receptor (sTfR) levels. Hum Mol Genet 2011; 20(5):1042–7.

84. Vilarino-Guell C, Farrer MJ, Lin SC. A genetic risk factor for periodic limb movements in sleep. N Engl J Med 2008;358:425–7.

85. Kemlink D, Polo O, Frauscher B, et al. Replication of restless legs syndrome loci in three European populations. J Med Genet 2009;46:315–8.

86. Reich DE, Lander ES. On the allelic spectrum of human disease. Trends Genet 2001;17:502–10.

87. Xiong L, Catoire H, Dion P, et al. MEIS1 intronic risk haplotype associated with restless legs syndrome affects its mRNA and protein expression levels. Hum Mol Genet 2009;18:1065–74.

88. Azcoitia V, Aracil M, Martinez AC, et al. The homeo-domain protein Meis1 is essential for definitive hematopoiesis and vascular patterning in the mouse embryo. Dev Biol 2005;280:307–20.

89. Manolio TA, Collins FS, Cox NJ, et al. Finding the missing heritability of complex diseases. Nature 2009;461:747–53.

90. Mardis ER. Next-generation DNA sequencing methods. Annu Rev Genomics Hum Genet 2008;9: 387–402.

91. Desautels A, Turecki G, Xiong L, et al. Mutational analysis of neurotensin in familial restless legs syndrome. Mov Disord 2004;19:90–4.

Genetics of Narcolepsy

Juliette Faraco, PhD, Emmanuel Mignot, MD, PhD*

KEYWORDS

- Narcolepsy • Genetics • Human leukocyte antigen
- Hypocretin • Orexin • Autoimmune

Narcolepsy is characterized by excessive daytime sleepiness, symptoms of dissociated rapid eye movement (REM) sleep (sleep paralysis, hypnagogic hallucinations), disrupted nocturnal sleep, and cataplexy (brief episodes of muscle weakness triggered by emotions). These symptoms all reflect a dysregulation of transitions between the states of wakefulness (daytime sleepiness, unconsolidated nocturnal sleep), non-REM (NREM) sleep, and REM sleep (sleep-onset REM periods, sleep paralysis, hallucinations, cataplexy). While most of these symptoms appear in the general population, particularly in the context of sleep deprivation or other sleep disorders, cataplexy is highly specific to narcolepsy. Onset is most often in childhood, peaking between 10 and 25 years of age, and once established the disease is lifelong. Recent work in humans and animal models has resulted in rapid and substantial progress in understanding the pathophysiology underlying narcolepsy.

HUMAN LEUKOCYTE ANTIGEN IN NARCOLEPSY

A strong association between narcolepsy and specific class II HLA antigens (DR2 and DQ1, 100% vs 30%) was first noted in the Japanese population.[1] HLA class II antigens are present on immune cells, and function to present processed foreign peptides to T cells by engaging the T-cell receptor. The initial association was rapidly confirmed in individuals of European descent.[2,3] DR2 and DQ1 are in complete disequilibrium in Japanese, but substantially less so in African Americans, and the association was found to be more variable in African Americans.[4] In Japanese and Europeans, the predisposing DQB1*0602 allele occurs together with DQA1*0102 on a haplotype with DRB1*1501. In African Americans, however, these DQB1 and DQA1 alleles are found with distinct DRB1 haplotypes, particularly DRB1*1503, DRB1*1501, DRB1*1101, and DRB1*0806.[5,6] Comparative high-resolution mapping among ethnic groups allowed refinement of the susceptibility region by examining the frequency of alternative haplotypes, demonstrating that DQB1*0602 is the most specific marker for narcolepsy in all ethnic groups.

The DQB1 and DQA1 loci (encoding DQβ and DQα, respectively) are located adjacent to each other within a 20-kb segment of the major histocompatibility complex (MHC) class II region on human chromosome 6. The translated products form a functional cell surface αβ heterodimer known as the HLA DQ antigen, which binds foreign or self antigens and presents these to the T-cell receptor to effect either an immune response or tolerance (**Fig. 1**). DQB1*0602 and DQA1*0102 are in nearly complete linkage disequilibrium in all populations, making it very difficult to study independent contributions of the two genes, or whether they are required to act together to confer narcolepsy susceptibility. DQA1*0102 occurs in conjunction with a variety of non-DQB1*0601 haplotypes, and these do not increase risk for narcolepsy, therefore DQA1*0102 by itself does not predispose to the disease. Although 90% of narcolepsy cases are associated with DQB1*0602, this is a common allele across ethnic groups, ranging from 12% in

Stanford Center for Sleep Sciences and Medicine, 1050 Arastradero Road, Building A, 2nd Floor, Palo Alto, CA 94304, USA
* Corresponding author.
E-mail address: mignot@stanford.edu

Sleep Med Clin 6 (2011) 217–228
doi:10.1016/j.jsmc.2011.03.001
1556-407X/11/$ – see front matter

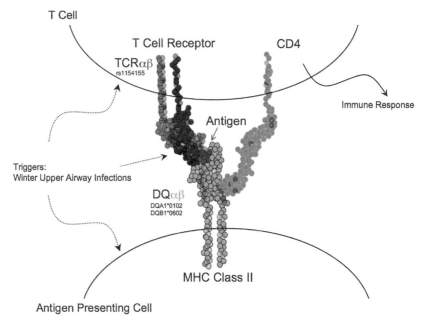

Fig. 1. The immunologic synapse in which class II major histocompatibility complex (MHC) DQ heterodimer presents antigen to the T-cell receptor on the responder T cell. The proportion of HLA DQA1*0102-DQB1*0602 heterodimers available to present a specific antigen is thought to modulate narcolepsy risk. T-cell receptor α variants in linkage with rs1154155 may confer risk by marking an amino acid variant or by influencing usage of a pathogenic J segment. Potential triggers include winter upper airway infections such as *Streptococcus pyogenes* or influenza A H1N1. These infections may yield antigens that stimulate an autoimmune response in conjunction with narcolepsy-associated MHC class II and T-cell receptor variants. Alternatively, they may activate dormant T-cell clones, or T-cell clones not appropriately deleted in the thymus; they may also act indirectly by increasing permeability of the blood-brain barrier.

Japanese to 38% in African Americans, and thus is not sufficient for the development of the disease.

It is also notable that the association with DQB1*0602 is particularly strong only in cases with typical cataplexy,[7,8] which in turn is also associated with low or undetectable cerebrospinal fluid (CSF) hypocretin-1, also known as orexin.[9] Indeed, less than 1% of cases with low hypocretin levels are DQB1*0602 negative. The HLA association is markedly decreased or absent in cases without cataplexy,[9] suggesting that disease heterogeneity is present among DQB1*0602-negative subjects and those without cataplexy.

Carriers of 2 HLA DQB1*0602 alleles (homozygotes) have an additional two- to fourfold risk for narcolepsy compared with heterozygotes, and may exhibit more severe symptoms,[10] thus the effect is not merely dominant/additive.[11–13] Other HLA alleles also modulate narcolepsy risk in DQB1*0602 heterozygotes. Large studies of narcolepsy-cataplexy patients and controls from multiple ethnic groups[11,12] identified numerous additional predisposing alleles including DQB1*0301, DQA1*06, DRB1*04, DRB1*08, DRB1*11, and DRB1*12. The most notable of these is DQB1*0301, which yields consistently high relative risks in all ethnic groups (**Table 1**). Surprisingly, the predisposing DQB1*0301 effect was noted in the context of a wide variety of DQA1 haplotypes. This finding could imply that the predisposing antigen-binding activity in this case is specified by unique variations encoded by DQB1*0301 and independent of those present on the DQα chain, or it may produce susceptibility in a mechanism independent of DQα-DQβ pairing altogether.[12]

Several protective alleles were also found to reach statistical significance: DQB1*0601, DQB1*0501, and DQA1*01 (non-DQA1*0102) (see **Table 1**). It is noteworthy that DQB1*0601 is protective but is structurally very similar to HLA DQB1*0602; this indicates that very minor changes in the peptide-binding pocket may determine disease risk. Moderate protective effects were also found for DQA1*0103-DQB1*0603,[11] more recently also reported through a genome-wide association (GWA) study in narcolepsy.[14] An emerging hypothesis regarding protective haplotypes is that part of the protective effect may be mediated through DQA1 and DQB1 alleles that have the ability to pair with DQA1*0102 and DQB1*0602. Two of the haplotypes with the strongest protective effects carry DQA1*01 alleles that

Table 1
Risks of HLA DQA1-DQB1 alleles carried in trans of DQB1*0602 in narcolepsy patients

DQA1-DQB1	Caucasians			African Americans			Japanese			Koreans			All Groups (Mantel Haenszel)			
	Narcolepsy n = 17	Control n = 255	OR	Narcolepsy n = 53	Control n = 397	OR	Narcolepsy n = 89	Control n = 1306	OR	Narcolepsy n = 77	Control n = 395	OR	Chi Square	P Value	OR	95% Interval
102-0602/x*-0301[a]	55	48	2.06	17	85	1.73	21	145	2.47	22	61	2.19	29.39	5.92^{-8}	2.08	1.60–1.72
102-0602/0101-0501	13	36	0.5	6	76	0.54	2	105	0.26	2	34	0.28	12.2	4.80^{-4}	0.43	0.27–0.69
102-0602/103-0601	0	4	0	0	4	0	8	297	0.33	1	48	0.1	18.54	1.70^{-5}	0.24	0.12–0.48
102-0602/103-0603[b]	3	15	0.29	2	19	0.78	0	7	0	0	2	0	3.71	.05	0.37	0.14–0.98
102-0602/other DQB1[c]	99	152	0.94	28	213	0.97	58	752	1.34	52	252	1.18	0.33	.56	1.08	0.85–1.37

Abbreviation: OR, odds ratio.

[a] x*-0301 includes DQA1*03, *05, *0601.

[b] Data replicated in Ref.[14]

[c] Includes DQB1*02, 0302, 0303, 0401, 0402, 0502, 0503, 0603, 0609.

Data from Mignot E, Lin L, Rogers W, et al. Complex HLA-DR and -DQ interactions confer risk of narcolepsy-cataplexy in three ethnic groups. Am J Hum Genet 2001;68:686–99; and Hong SC, Lin L, Lo B, et al. DQB1*0301 and DQB1*0601 modulate narcolepsy susceptibility in Koreans. Hum Immunol 2007;68:59–68.

are non-DQA1*0102, namely DQA1*0103 (with DQB1*0601) and DQA1*0101 (with DQB1*0501).[12] In vitro studies have shown that structurally similar DQα and DQβ chains (eg, those from the same family, such as DQ1) can form stable *trans*-heterodimers.[15] Thus DQB1*05 and DQB1*06 can form heterodimers with DQA1*01 subtypes, but not other DQA1 alleles (all these alleles belong to the large group DQ1). These haplotypes may therefore exert a protective effect by reducing the incidence of the pathogenic DQA1*0102-DQB1*0602 heterodimer through pairing the *trans*-located DQA1*01, non-DQA1*0102 allele with DQB1*0602. Such *trans* effects have been documented in two other HLA-associated autoimmune diseases: celiac disease[16] and type 1 diabetes.[17]

HLA ASSOCIATIONS AND AUTOIMMUNITY

The interaction of HLA proteins with processed antigens determines the resulting immune response. Associations of class II MHC antigens have been well characterized in a variety of autoimmune diseases, although narcolepsy, with the nearly ubiquitous association with a single DQB1 allele, shows the tightest of any such interactions (reviewed in Ref.[18]).

The tight association with DQB1*0602, typical peripubertal onset, and the low concordance in monozygotic twins all suggest an autoimmune mechanism for narcolepsy, but certain features have been noted to be less consistent with a typical autoimmune mechanism (eg, females are not at increased risk), and attempts over many years failed to detect direct evidence for humoral or cellular immunity (no specific autoantibodies, disease not transferred through injection of serum into mice, no differences in activity of T cells and natural killer [NK] cells in narcolepsy cases[18–20]). In 2010, reactive autoantibodies against the Tribbles 2 homolog (Trib2) were identified in narcolepsy sera,[21] a finding replicated by two groups.[22,23] Anti-TRIB2 antibodies were noted to be most prevalent soon after narcolepsy onset, with detected antibodies and titer levels dropping sharply within 2 to 3 years of cataplexy onset. Autoantibodies were prevalent among DQB1*0602-positive cases with cataplexy (ranging from 14% to 26% in the 3 studies), but rare in cases without cataplexy or normal controls (including DQB1*0602-positive controls; identified in 2%–4% of controls). This finding represents the first replicated direct evidence of an autoimmune process in narcolepsy, but it is not clear how the identified antibodies relate to the disease process, as there is no direct evidence that the antibodies injure hypocretin neurons. TRIB2 is also widely expressed in brain and other tissues, but cell loss in narcolepsy appears to be highly specific to hypocretin neurons. Alternative models of the role of these antibodies have been proposed[24]; for example, hypocretin cell death by another cause could release intracellular TRIB2 protein, leading to the production of autoantibodies (epitope spreading), or an inflammatory response could independently lead to hypocretin cell death and to the production of TRIB2 antibodies.

PREVALENCE AND HERITABILITY

In the general population, narcolepsy-cataplexy occurs with a fairly consistent prevalence of approximately 0.02% in various Caucasian groups, with a lower prevalence in Israeli Jews (0.002%), and a somewhat higher prevalence in Japanese (0.16%) and individuals of African descent.[25,26] These prevalence rates also partially correspond with higher frequency of DQB1*0602 in African Americans (38%) and lower frequency in Ashkenazi Jews (3%–6%), although not in Japanese (12%). The prevalence of narcolepsy without cataplexy is largely unknown and is difficult to ascertain. Patients are likely to be underdiagnosed or misdiagnosed, and the diagnosis, including presence of sleep-onset REM periods (SOREMPs), lacks specificity. Population-based studies indicate that 1% to 3% of the population report sleepiness with multiple SOREMPs detected by multiple sleep latency testing.[27,28]

Until recently narcolepsy was considered to be a familial disorder, and familial occurrence of narcolepsy-cataplexy was reported in the initial 1887 report by Westphal.[29] On reexamination, it is clear that many previously reported instances of familial occurrence represent unrecognized obstructive sleep apnea in family members, and that narcolepsy is primarily a sporadic disorder, albeit one with a strong genetic basis for susceptibility. Familial clustering occurs, with 8% to 10% of patients reporting another family member with narcolepsy-cataplexy. These first-degree relatives have an overall risk of 0.9% to 2.3%, which is low, but represents a 10- to 40-fold higher risk than the general population.[18,25] Increased rates of excessive sleepiness and isolated REM sleep abnormalities (hypnagogic hallucinations, sleep paralysis) have also been reported in first-degree relatives,[25] but overall risk is difficult to quantify because of the high prevalence of excessive daytime sleepiness in the general population.

Non-HLA genes also clearly contribute to susceptibility, as the relative risk observed in first-degree relatives is much greater than can be explained by the effect of HLA.[11] Multiplex families in which the disease is transmitted across multiple generations have been reported, but are rare (see Ref.[25]). It is notable that a significant proportion of these multiplex families (30%) show no association with HLA DQB1*0602. As these families are both rare and small in size, gene identification through linkage studies has been precluded.

Studies of monozygotic twins with narcolepsy-cataplexy show a low concordance rate. Twenty-five percent of previously reported monozygotic twins (21 case reports) are concordant for narcolepsy-cataplexy (32% concordance when narcolepsy either with or without cataplexy is considered).[25] It is noteworthy that only 3 of 5 concordant twin pairs that were HLA tested (60%) were found to be DQB1*0602 positive, consistent with lower rates of DQB1*0602 positivity among multiplex family cases. These findings underline a role for high-penetrance non-HLA genes in genetic susceptibility in these cases, as well as the requirement for environmental triggers acting on a susceptible genetic background to initiate disease.

POTENTIAL ENVIRONMENTAL TRIGGERS

Recent studies indicate that upper airway infections may act to trigger narcolepsy. Several studies have noted increased levels of streptococcal antibodies (antistreptolysin O) in narcolepsy patients within 3 years of onset versus age-matched controls, but not in cases with long-standing disease.[22,30,31] Narcolepsy was also more common among people reporting a diagnosis of strep throat before the age of 21 years.[32] Emerging evidence also suggests that exposure to the H1N1 subtype of influenza A virus, particularly through exposure to H1N1 vaccine formulated with adjuvant, may also be a rare trigger for disease development. In the period September 2009 to August 2010, an apparent increase in recent-onset narcolepsy cases was noted in major narcolepsy centers in France, Canada, and the United States.[33] Of 31 cases identified (at Stanford, Montpellier, and Montreal) and studied for past H1N1 exposure or vaccination, 14 developed disease between 2 and 8 weeks of H1N1 vaccination, and of these, 11 received vaccine formulated with adjuvant system 03 (AS03). Two cases developed disease following documented or likely H1N1 viral infection. All were DQB1*0602 positive, with definite cataplexy, and documented hypocretin-1 deficiency (<100 pg/mL in CSF) in 10 cases. Several clinical features were notable, including rapid disease development of both severe sleepiness and severe cataplexy, as well as atypical age at onset (5 cases older than 38 and 2 cases younger than 5 years). In addition, 11 postvaccination cases showed high antistreptolysin O titers, suggesting recent or recurrent streptococcal infections as previously noted, but none had detectable anti-TRIB2 antibodies. These results indicate that streptococcal antigens and/or H1N1 antigens could potentially trigger narcolepsy in predisposed individuals. Individuals with anti TRIB2 antibodies may also represent a different subset of triggering factors.

The highly constrained DQB1 and T-cell receptor (TCR) sequences involved suggest that an important peptide antigen acts as a specific trigger (see above). In this context *Streptococcus*, H1N1, or other factors could be acting as nonspecific immune triggers, for example, *Streptococcus* infection could lead to superantigen stimulation of dormant autoreactive T-cell clones. Likewise, in the case of H1N1 the strength of immune response may be more important than the specificity (adjuvant-formulated vaccine is associated with a stronger immune response). Both factors could also potentially act indirectly by increasing blood-brain penetration.

ANIMAL MODELS OF NARCOLEPSY

Narcolepsy has been reported in a variety of species, and reports of narcolepsy-cataplexy in dogs led to the establishment of a canine narcolepsy colony at Stanford in the 1970s. Breeding and backcrossing of narcoleptic dogs of a variety of breeds indicated that as in humans, canine narcolepsy is most frequently sporadic and is not transmitted as a simple Mendelian trait. In 1977 several affected Dobermans, including 2 from the same litter, and several affected Labrador retrievers were found to carry autosomal recessive mutations causing narcolepsy-cataplexy, leading to the establishment of the canine genetic model for the disease.[34] In both the sporadic and genetic forms, dogs exhibited pronounced cataplexy triggered by food or play, and showed decreased bout length for sleep and wake compared with matched controls. Animals also showed short sleep and REM latency, underscoring the similarity of canine narcolepsy to the human disorder. An extensive positional cloning project identified mutations the hypocretin receptor 2 gene (HCRTR2) causing the disorder in Dobermans and Labradors, as well as in a family of Dachshunds.[35] The 3 identified mutations all caused severe changes (exon skipping leading to frameshift and premature stop; loss of ligand binding by the receptor), loss of function in the encoded protein and, therefore, impairment of postsynaptic hypocretin neurotransmission.

In parallel with the canine molecular studies, investigators initiated a variety of genetic models to study the biology of the same neuropeptide system, but under the name Orexin. The single ligand gene encodes 2 highly related peptides, released by proteolytic cleavage and termed hypocretin-1 and hypocretin-2, or alternately orexins A and B. These peptides then signal two related G-protein–coupled receptors alternately called hypocretin/orexin receptors 1 and 2.[36,37] Several rodent models have been developed to study the hypocretin/orexin system in detail. Chemelli and colleagues[38] first described a narcolepsy-like phenotype in orexin knockout mice, which were initially created under the hypothesis that the primary role of the neuropeptides was to stimulate appetite (thus "orexin").

Expecting the animals to have reduced appetite and decreased body weight, these investigators were surprised to find that orexin knockout mice primarily displayed sleep/wake state fragmentation and behavioral arrests, similar to cataplexy in humans and narcoleptic canines. Further studies examined the distinct effects of loss of orexin/hypocretin-containing cells as opposed to selective loss of the neuropeptide itself,[39] first in mice and later in rats.[40] These animals carried a transgene with the hypocretin gene promoter driving expression of an expanded polyglutamine repeat from the ataxin-3 gene, leading to selective degeneration of hypocretin neurons by 12 weeks of age. Initial studies indicated that cell ablation in these transgenic mice led to late-onset obesity despite them eating less than nontransgenic littermates.[39] Later studies revealed a more complex basis to the metabolic disruption involving genetic background as well as sex-based differences. The phenotype was studied on a homogeneous background to determine the relative influence of known strain-based metabolic differences, versus selective loss of hypocretin/orexin transmission or loss of hypocretin/orexin cells including coexpressed peptides and neuromodulators.[41] Ligand knockout mice did not significantly gain weight compared with wild type when compared on the same background. However, Ataxin-3 transgenic mice had more weight gain, potentially resulting from concomitant loss of other neurotransmitters in the ablated cells (ie, loss of glutamatergic signaling of same cells, loss of neuronal activity–regulated pentraxin, and dynorphin transmission). Further studies[42] identified sex-based differences in these metabolic changes not seen in previous studies that were restricted to male mice. Body weight gain became pronounced in female knockout mice compared with wild-type littermates, but this was not clear in males. The same pattern was observed in transgenic cell-ablated animals. Finally, it was also noted that because hypocretin/

orexin-deficient mice have reduced wake-bout length, and normal mice typically wait a few minutes after waking up from sleep to eat, reduced food intake could be secondary to sleep-wake disturbances.[43] Overall, these studies suggest that the loss of hypocretin/orexin disrupts appetite and energy homeostasis, but that these effects are variable and could be very indirectly mediated. These observations are in line with those in humans, in whom the development of narcolepsy is often, but not always, associated with weight gain, notably in children.

Additional models lacking the two hypocretin/orexin receptor proteins were created.[44] Mice with targeted disruption of both receptors (double knockout) had a phenotype resembling the ligand knockout animals. By contrast, receptor-2–deficient mice showed similar phenotypes in terms of fragmentation of sleep and wakefulness, but the receptor-2–deficient mice had a milder phenotype with less frequent cataplexy-like attacks and transitions from wake to REM or non-REM to REM sleep compared with mice lacking the ligand. By contrast, hypocretin receptor-1 knockout animals had no phenotype or perhaps slight sleep fragmentation abnormalities, suggesting a more minor role in the expression of the narcolepsy phenotype.

HYPOCRETIN DEFICIENCY IN NARCOLEPSY

The study of narcolepsy in canines led to our current understanding of the disease pathophysiology. As in humans, most cases of canine narcolepsy are sporadic and genetically complex, but the identification of dog pedigrees segregating an autosomal recessive form of narcolepsy with clear-cut cataplexy led to identification of mutations of HCRTR2 as the basis of the disease.[35] Subsequent studies quickly led to an understanding of the basis of the disease in humans, identifying a profound reduction in hypocretin gene expression and peptide content in postmortem narcoleptic brains, and low or undetectable levels of hypocretin-1 in the CSF of narcolepsy cases.[45–47] Mutation screening of the hypocretin ligand and receptor genes in narcolepsy cases was performed focusing on rare DQB1*0602-negative and familial cases, which would be more likely to carry mutations. A single mutation was identified in a case of early-onset narcolepsy with cataplexy present at 6 months.[46] The mutation introduced a highly charged arginine residue into the signal peptide of the prepro-hypocretin protein. Functional analysis suggested abnormal trafficking of the mutant peptide precursor, resulting in toxicity to the cells, supported by undetectable hypocretin in the CSF. Further studies, based both on candidate gene sequencing and GWA design, have been performed in samples of European and Japanese ancestry, but have failed to find mutations in or single-nucleotide polymorphism (SNP) associations with the hypocretin system genes in more typical cases of sporadic DQB1*0602-positive narcolepsy.[46,48–51] Therefore, although narcolepsy-cataplexy is clearly associated with deficient hypocretin neurotransmission, this is not due to hypocretin gene mutations or variants. It is interesting that no hypocretin receptor 2 mutations have yet been identified in humans, whereas 3 distinct mutations have been identified in dogs with a typical narcolepsy-cataplexy phenotype. The reasons for this dichotomy are unclear, but may reflect species differences in upregulation of cholinergic systems, leading to expression of cataplexy that are a result of deficient hypocretin transmission.[34,52] Narcoleptic dogs with hypocretin receptor 2 mutations display typical cataplexy, but mice lacking HCRTR2 exhibit less cataplexy than hypocretin/orexin ligand knockout mice, or mice lacking both receptors.[44] It may thus be that HCRTR2 mutations in humans result in a diminished phenotype. The pattern of highly selective hypocretin cell loss together with the lack of identified mutations again points to an underlying autoimmune disease mechanism. Although hypocretin is only one of several neurotransmitters implicated in sleep regulation, it is notable that only deficiency in hypocretin leads to such a highly specific sleep-related phenotype.

NON-HLA, NON-HCRT GENES IN NARCOLEPSY

Several studies have attempted to map narcolepsy genes in human families through linkage,[53,54] but regions of suggested linkage have not been replicated. More recently efforts have focused on GWA studies using high-density SNP platforms, with 3 such studies published to date (**Table 2**). Miyagawa and colleagues[50] examined associations in a set of 222 narcolepsy versus 389 Japanese controls, and replication in 159 narcolepsy versus 190 controls. In each round, the smallest P value at rs5770917, a SNP located between CPT1B and CHKB, ranged from 1 to 6 $\times$ 10^{-4} (odds ratio [OR] = 1.79). Additional genotyping in small samples of Koreans, European Americans, and African Americans showed differences in minor allele frequencies in the same direction, but reached significance only in Koreans (P = .03, 115 cases, 309 controls). Of note, this SNP had very unfavorable minor allele frequencies in Caucasian (4%) and African American (2.6%) controls, underscoring the wide-ranging differences in allele frequencies among different populations. Subsequent GWA studies found no association of this SNP in individuals of European descent,[14,51] but an association (P = 3.6 $\times$ 10^{-3}, OR = 1.56, irrespective of HLA haplotype) was noted in a Japanese sample of essential hypersomnia (EHS; 137 cases, 569 controls), a heterogeneous disorder also showing an increased association with DQB1*0602, and thus potentially including cases with incomplete presentation of the narcolepsy-cataplexy phenotype.[50] CPT1B, a rate-limiting enzyme in long-chain fatty acid β-oxidation in muscle mitochondria, and CHKB, a kinase involved in phosphatidylcholine synthesis, are both plausible candidates in terms of modulation of narcolepsy and REM sleep effects.

A larger GWA primarily focused on individuals of European descent from North America and Europe

Table 2
Non-HLA narcolepsy susceptibility loci

Gene	Reported SNP	Comments
CPT1B/CHKB	rs5770917	Identified in Japanese, replicated in Koreans, not significant in European or African descent. Loci have roles in β-oxidation and phosphatidylcholine synthesis, potentially modulating REM
TCRA	rs1154155	Identified in Caucasians, replicated across ethnic groups. Independently replicated in Europeans and Japanese with OR-positive essential hypersomnia. Potential linkage with variant causing biased J-segment usage or amino acid change
DQA2	rs2858884	Identified in Europeans. Not replicated in an independent sample of European descent. SNP in linkage disequilibrium with protective DRBl*1301-DQA1*0103-DQB1*0603
P2RY11	rs2305795	Identified in Europeans, with replication across ethnic groups. Not yet replicated independently. Immunomodulatory function/reduced ATP-induced apoptosis of some immune cells

Abbreviations: ATP, adenosine triphosphate; SNP, single-nucleotide polymorphism.

identified a different SNP variant strongly associated with narcolepsy across 3 ethnic groups.[51] In a sample of 807 Caucasian narcolepsy cases versus 1074 HLA-DQB1*0602-positive controls, 3 SNPs within the T-cell receptor α (TCRA) locus were significantly associated, with highest significance across racial groups at rs1154155 within the J-segment region ($P = 1.9 \times 10^{-13}$, OR = 1.87; 807 cases, 1174 controls). This SNP showed significant association on replication in Caucasians ($P = 3.67 \times 10^{-5}$, 363 cases, 355 controls) and Asians (from Japan and Korea, 561 cases, 605 controls, $P = 2.30 \times 10^{-7}$), and similar OR but not reaching significance in a small set of African Americans, in whom the allele is uncommon (133 cases, 144 controls, $P = .39$, allele frequency 10% in cases, 8% in controls). The population attributable risk for rs1154155C in Caucasians is estimated to be 20%, but is 43% in Asians, who have a much higher allele frequency, potentially explaining increased prevalence of narcolepsy in Japan, despite lower DQB1*0602 frequency.[11] An additional study in Europeans also replicated the finding in DRB1*1501-positive (presumed DQB1*0602+) cases and controls (discovery + replication $P = 5.3 \times 10^{-7}$, 932 cases, 1449 controls, OR = 1.54).[14] The same SNP was studied in the Japanese EHS sample, and was found to be significantly increased among patients who carried HLA-DRB1*1501-DQB1*0602 versus HLA-matched controls ($P = .008$, 47 cases, 151 controls), but showed no signal among those that were HLA negative.[55] This finding suggests that the portion of EHS that is HLA-DRB1*1501-DQB1*0602-positive shares a similar genetic basis and autoimmune pathophysiology with narcolepsy-cataplexy, representing an incompletely penetrant phenotype. This result is also suggested by increased DQB1*0602 frequency in narcolepsy without cataplexy cases, which are typically approximately 30% to 40% positive (vs 25% in controls), suggesting that approximately 5% to 15% of these cases have a hypocretin-related pathology, a figure also consistent with CSF hypocretin-1 studies in this subgroup of patients.

The homogeneity of OR and strong replication in independent samples of multiple ethnic groups indicate that the TCRA is a significant and general susceptibility factor for narcolepsy. The TCRA locus is a logical biological candidate, as it encodes the α chain of the mature T-cell receptor αβ heterodimer that is localized on the surface of T cells and recognizes antigens bound and presented by class I or class II MHC molecules (such as DQ described earlier, see **Fig. 1**). Following engagement with the antigen-MHC complex, the T-cell receptor initiates immune response through activation of at least 3 families of transcription factors: nuclear factor of activated

T cells (NFAT), activating protein 1 (AP-1), and nuclear factor κB (NF-κB).[56] Like the immunoglobulin loci, the TCRA locus undergoes somatic cell recombination, which occurs between 46 functional variable (V) and 49 functional joining (J) segments. Precisely how a J-segment region polymorphism (rs1154155C or another variant in tight linkage disequilibrium) could increase the risk of narcolepsy is unknown, but could involve nonrandom VJα choices in recombination. As narcolepsy is almost entirely associated with a single HLA allele, it may be hypothesized that the DQ1 heterodimer antigen encoded by DQB1*0602/DQA1*0102 could interact with a TCR idiotype representing a specific VJα recombinant associated with the presence of rs1154155 (directly or indirectly). This finding indicates that it is all but certain that narcolepsy is an autoimmune disease as, unlike HLA, functional TCRs are only expressed in immune T cells. In the context of a selected antigenic trigger, this could then lead to further immune reaction ending in the destruction of hypocretin-producing cells.

Finally, another large GWA studied narcolepsy-cataplexy cases and controls from Europe, and used the process of imputation to infer genotypes at untyped SNP markers. SNP rs2858884, located upstream of the DQA2 locus, was associated with narcolepsy in a DRB1*1501-matched discovery sample ($P = 4.65 \times 10^{-5}$, OR = 2.1, 562 cases, 702 controls) and replication sample ($P = .038$, OR = 1.4, 370 cases, 495 controls).[14] The associated allele was more common in controls than in cases, indicating a protective effect, which was found to be explained partially by linkage disequilibrium with DRB1*1301-DQB1*0603. This DQ variant differs by only 2 amino acids from DQB1*0602, and in the context of DRB1*1301 is carried together with DQA1*0103, a haplotype with known protective effects, potentially through DQA1*0103 *trans*-pairing with DQB1*0602.[11,12]

An additional candidate locus was identified through screening and replication of second-tier significance hits in the Hallmayer GWA study of European and North American narcolepsy cases and controls. SNP marker rs4804122, a marker located in a region of high linkage disequilibrium spanning the PPAN through DNMT1 loci on chromosome 19, was associated with narcolepsy ($P = 5.92 \times 10^{-5}$, OR 0.76, 788 cases, 1061 controls). The SNP association with narcolepsy was strongly replicated in Caucasian cases and controls ($P = 5.4 \times 10^{-4}$, OR = 0.77; 603 cases, 907 controls) but was not significant in a large sample of Asian cases and controls. Comparison of regional linkage disequilibrium suggested alternative markers that could be associated across ethnic groups, and SNP rs2305795, located in the 3′ untranslated region of the P2RY11 purinergic receptor gene, showed the highest association with narcolepsy across 3 ethnic groups ($P = 6.14 \times 10^{-10}$, OR 0.78; 2522 cases, 3167 controls).[57] Little is known about the function of this particular purinergic receptor, as the Y11 form is present as a pseudogene in rodents, although in humans it is widely expressed, with pronounced levels in the brain and in white blood cells.[58] Purinergic signaling plays a fundamental role in immune regulation, modulating proliferation, chemotaxis, and apoptosis in a variety of lymphoid cell types. Functional studies indicate that P2RY11 is expressed in $CD8^+$ T cells and NK cells, and that the A allele of rs2305795 is associated with reduced P2RY11 expression in selected cell populations, and is also associated with reduced ATP-induced apoptosis of immune cells. Thus this locus could affect susceptibility to narcolepsy through a variety of mechanisms, including modulation of immune response to an infectious trigger, modulation of an autoimmune process, and mediation of neutrophil chemotaxis, or potentially have direct apoptotic effects on hypocretin cells.

SECONDARY NARCOLEPSY IN OTHER GENETIC DISORDERS

Although cataplexy is highly selective and almost pathognomonic for narcolepsy, it has also been reported in patients with other known genetic diseases. Niemann-Pick disease type C (NPC) is a recessive lysosomal storage disorder. Approximately 95% of cases are due to recessive mutations in the NPC1 integral membrane protein, with another 5% due to mutations in the NPC2 locus, a secreted cholesterol binding protein. Both proteins are involved in cholesterol efflux from late endosomes/lysosomes.[59] Clinical symptoms and severity are variable, but include hepatosplenomegaly and neurologic findings, including abnormalities of the electroencephalogram during sleep.[60] CSF hypocretin-1 levels in NPC are repeatedly found to be significantly lower than in controls, although never in the very low sporadic narcolepsy range, suggesting that the lysosomal storage abnormalities affect the function or viability of hypocretin-producing cells in the hypothalamus. Norrie disease is primarily an X-linked eye disease causing childhood blindness due to degeneration of the neuroretina, but other clinical features are variably present depending on the size of the underlying chromosomal deletion, which can include deletion of the monoamine oxidase loci. Cataplexy and REM sleep abnormalities have been described in Norrie disease in association with absent monoamine oxidase activity and increased serotonin levels.[61] Narcolepsy-like symptoms including excessive daytime sleepiness, REM sleep abnormalities, and cataplexy have also been reported in Prader-Willi syndrome (PWS),[62,63] an imprinting-related disorder caused by maternal uniparental disomy of chromosome 15q11-q12, or alternatively, deletion/disruption of paternal copies of the corresponding loci. PWS is characterized by obesity, muscular hypotonia, mental retardation, short stature, and hypogonadotropic hypogonadism. Several studies have reported reduced CSF hypocretin levels.[64] These results indicate that the excessive sleepiness seen in PWS is not simply secondary to hypoventilation and obstructive sleep apnea in these obese individuals, but rather suggests a central hypothalamic dysfunction.

Familial narcolepsy has also been reported in conjunction with cerebellar ataxia and deafness.[65] A multigeneration family from Sweden segregated an autosomal dominant syndrome including cerebellar ataxia with sensorineural deafness. Four of 5 affected individuals also had narcolepsy with cataplexy. Subjects also showed enlargement of the third ventricle, atrophy of the cerebellum and cerebral hemispheres, and loss of olivary bulges.[66] CSF level of HCRT-1 was tested in one affected member (DQB1*0602 negative) and found to be 97.0 pg/mL, below the diagnostic threshold for narcolepsy (<110 pg/mL), suggesting partial loss of HCRT cells and/or disruption of projection fields in the disorder.[67] Familial narcolepsy with an otherwise normal neurologic examination but with degenerative changes of the substantia nigra has also been reported in a large multiplex pedigree (5 generations) with 2 individuals with narcolepsy-cataplexy and an additional 7 meeting the International Classification of Sleep Disorders criteria for narcolepsy but without cataplexy.[68] Indeed collateral damage to hypocretinergic cells is not uncommon in Parkinson disease, and may underlie some nonmotor symptoms of that disease such as excessive daytime sleepiness.[69]

SUMMARY

Significant strides have recently been made in understanding narcolepsy, which can now formally be considered an autoimmune disease based on the identification of strong predisposing genetic variants within the HLA and T-cell receptor loci, as well as the identification of increased levels of specific autoantibodies near disease onset. Progress has also been made toward identifying antigenic triggers of the autoimmune process. These recent findings are consistent with previous genetic results suggesting complex genetics requiring environmental triggers to act on a susceptible (DQB1*0602 positive) background, or more rarely, the action of more highly penetrant gene variants acting through a DQB1*0602-independent mechanism (as in concordant monozygotic twins, or multiplex families). Only in rare cases have these highly penetrant genes been identified, as in the single detected HCRT mutation, and more commonly are yet unidentified or are associated with additional strong neurologic phenotypes (such as NPC, or narcolepsy-ataxia-deafness). These non-HLA/non-HCRT narcolepsy loci are likely to be identified in the future through whole genome sequencing, or exome sequencing studies of rare families, and may prove to have modulatory effects on the presentation of the more prevalent autoimmune narcolepsy phenotype. Additional susceptibility loci (such as P2RY11) are already emerging and are under active study regarding influence on immune function. Recent strides in the genetics of other autoimmune diseases are pointing to the combined effects of clusters of immune-related susceptibility genes (often delineating immune pathways of significance for the disease), and these should be studied in the context of narcolepsy.[70–72] Variants at HLA DQ, TCRA, and other susceptibility loci may also prove to be useful in the identification of phenotypic subsets in more heterogeneous disorders such as narcolepsy without cataplexy and hypersomnias, as has been done for essential hypersomnia, which are likely to share overlapping pathophysiology.

REFERENCES

1. Juji T, Satake M, Honda Y, et al. HLA antigens in Japanese patients with narcolepsy. All the patients were DR2 positive. Tissue Antigens 1984;24:316–9.

2. Marcadet A, Gebuhrer L, Betuel H, et al. DNA polymorphism related to HLA-DR2 Dw2 in patients with narcolepsy. Immunogenetics 1985;22:679–83.

3. Mueller-Eckhardt G, Strohmaier P, Schendel DJ, et al. Possible male segregation distortion of DR2 haplotypes in narcolepsy patients. Hum Immunol 1987;20:189–93.

4. Neely S, Rosenberg R, Spire JP, et al. HLA antigens in narcolepsy. Neurology 1987;37:1858–60.

5. Matsuki K, Grumet FC, Lin X, et al. DQ (rather than DR) gene marks susceptibility to narcolepsy. Lancet 1992;339:1052.

6. Mignot E, Kimura A, Lattermann A, et al. Extensive HLA class II studies in 58 non-DRB1*15 (DR2) narcoleptic patients with cataplexy. Tissue Antigens 1997;49:329–41.

7. Matsuki K, Honda Y, Juji T. Diagnostic criteria for narcolepsy and HLA-DR2 frequencies. Tissue Antigens 1987;30:155–60.

8. Mignot E, Hayduk R, Black J, et al. HLA DQB1*0602 is associated with cataplexy in 509 narcoleptic patients. Sleep 1997;20:1012–20.

9. Lin L, Mignot E. Human leukocyte antigen and narcolepsy: present status and relationship with familial history and hypocretin deficiency. In: Bassetti C, Billiard M, Mignot E, editors. Narcolepsy and hypersomnia. New York: Informa Healthcare; 2007. p. 411–26 London.

10. Pelin Z, Guilleminault C, Risch N, et al. HLA-DQB1*0602 homozygosity increases relative risk for narcolepsy but not disease severity in two ethnic groups. US Modafinil in Narcolepsy Multicenter Study Group. Tissue Antigens 1998;51:96–100.

11. Mignot E, Lin L, Rogers W, et al. Complex HLA-DR and -DQ interactions confer risk of narcolepsy-cataplexy in three ethnic groups. Am J Hum Genet 2001;68:686–99.

12. Hong SC, Lin L, Lo B, et al. DQB1*0301 and DQB1*0601 modulate narcolepsy susceptibility in Koreans. Hum Immunol 2007;68:59–68.

13. Watson NF, Ton TG, Koepsell TD, et al. Does narcolepsy symptom severity vary according to HLA-DQB1*0602 allele status? Sleep 2010;33:29–35.

14. Hor H, Kutalik Z, Dauvilliers Y, et al. Genome-wide association study identifies new HLA class II haplotypes strongly protective against narcolepsy. Nat Genet 2010;42:786–9.

15. Kwok WW, Kovats S, Thurtle P, et al. HLA-DQ allelic polymorphisms constrain patterns of class II heterodimer formation. J Immunol 1993;150:2263–72.

16. Margaritte-Jeannin P, Babron MC, Bourgey M, et al. HLA-DQ relative risks for coeliac disease in European populations: a study of the European Genetics Cluster on Coeliac Disease. Tissue Antigens 2004; 63:562–7.

17. Koeleman BP, Lie BA, Undlien DE, et al. Genotype effects and epistasis in type 1 diabetes and HLA-DQ trans dimer associations with disease. Genes Immun 2004;5:381–8.

18. Chabas D, Taheri S, Renier C, et al. The genetics of narcolepsy. Annu Rev Genomics Hum Genet 2003; 4:459–83.

19. Overeem S, Verschuuren JJ, Fronczek R, et al. Immunohistochemical screening for autoantibodies against lateral hypothalamic neurons in human narcolepsy. J Neuroimmunol 2006;174:187–91.

20. Scammell TE. The frustrating and mostly fruitless search for an autoimmune cause of narcolepsy. Sleep 2006;29:601–2.

21. Cvetkovic-Lopes V, Bayer L, Dorsaz S, et al. Elevated Tribbles homolog 2-specific antibody levels in narcolepsy patients. J Clin Invest 2010;120:713–9.

22. Kawashima M, Lin L, Tanaka S, et al. Anti-Tribbles homolog 2 (TRIB2) autoantibodies in narcolepsy are associated with recent onset of cataplexy. Sleep 2010;33:869–74.

23. Toyoda H, Tanaka S, Miyagawa T, et al. Anti-Tribbles homolog 2 autoantibodies in Japanese patients with narcolepsy. Sleep 2010;33:875–8.

24. Lim AS, Scammell TE. The trouble with Tribbles: do antibodies against TRIB2 cause narcolepsy? Sleep 2010;33:857–8.

25. Mignot E. Genetic and familial aspects of narcolepsy. Neurology 1998;50:S16–22.

26. Longstreth WT Jr, Ton TG, Koepsell T, et al. Prevalence of narcolepsy in King County, Washington, USA. Sleep Med 2009;10:422–6.

27. Mignot E, Lin L, Finn L, et al. Correlates of sleep-onset REM periods during the Multiple Sleep Latency Test in community adults. Brain 2006;129:1609–23.

28. Singh M, Drake CL, Roth T. The prevalence of multiple sleep-onset REM periods in a population-based sample. Sleep 2006;29:890–5.

29. Schenck CH, Bassetti CL, Arnulf I, et al. English translations of the first clinical reports on narcolepsy and cataplexy by Westphal and Gelineau in the late 19th century, with commentary. J Clin Sleep Med 2007;3:301–11.

30. Billiard M, Laberti M, Reygrobellet C, et al. Elevated antibodies to streptococcal antigens in narcoleptic subjects. Sleep Res 1989;18:201.

31. Aran A, Lin L, Nevsimalova S, et al. Elevated anti-streptococcal antibodies in patients with recent narcolepsy onset. Sleep 2009;32:979–83.

32. Koepsell TD, Longstreth WT, Ton TG. Medical exposures in youth and the frequency of narcolepsy with cataplexy: a population-based case-control study in genetically predisposed people. J Sleep Res 2010;19:80–6.

33. Dauvilliers Y, Montplaisir J, Cochen V, et al. Post H1N1 narcolepsy-cataplexy. Sleep 2010;33:1428–30.

34. Nishino S. Clinical and neurobiological aspects of narcolepsy. Sleep Med 2007;8:373–99.

35. Lin L, Faraco J, Li R, et al. The sleep disorder canine narcolepsy is caused by a mutation in the hypocretin (orexin) receptor 2 gene. Cell 1999;98:365–76.

36. Sakurai T, Amemiya A, Ishii M, et al. Orexins and orexin receptors: a family of hypothalamic neuropeptides and G protein-coupled receptors that regulate feeding behavior. Cell 1998;92:573–85.

37. de Lecea L, Kilduff TS, Peyron C, et al. The hypocretins: hypothalamus-specific peptides with neuroexcitatory activity. Proc Natl Acad Sci U S A 1998;95:322–7.

38. Chemelli RM, Willie JT, Sinton CM, et al. Narcolepsy in orexin knockout mice: molecular genetics of sleep regulation. Cell 1999;98:437–51.

39. Hara J, Beuckmann CT, Nambu T, et al. Genetic ablation of orexin neurons in mice results in narcolepsy, hypophagia, and obesity. Neuron 2001;30:345–54.

40. Beuckmann CT, Sinton CM, Williams SC, et al. Expression of a poly-glutamine-ataxin-3 transgene in orexin neurons induces narcolepsy-cataplexy in the rat. J Neurosci 2004;24:4469–77.

41. Hara J, Yanagisawa M, Sakurai T. Difference in obesity phenotype between orexin-knockout mice and orexin neuron-deficient mice with same genetic background and environmental conditions. Neurosci Lett 2005;380:239–42.

42. Fujiki N, Yoshida Y, Zhang S, et al. Sex difference in body weight gain and leptin signaling in hypocretin/orexin deficient mouse models. Peptides 2006;27:2326–31.

43. Zhang S, Zeitzer JM, Sakurai T, et al. Sleep/wake fragmentation disrupts metabolism in a mouse model of narcolepsy. J Physiol 2007;581:649–63.

44. Willie JT, Chemelli RM, Sinton CM, et al. Distinct narcolepsy syndromes in Orexin receptor-2 and Orexin null mice: molecular genetic dissection of non-REM and REM sleep regulatory processes. Neuron 2003;38:715–30.

45. Nishino S, Ripley B, Overeem S, et al. Hypocretin (orexin) deficiency in human narcolepsy. Lancet 2000;355:39–40.

46. Peyron C, Faraco J, Rogers W, et al. A mutation in a case of early onset narcolepsy and a generalized absence of hypocretin peptides in human narcoleptic brains. Nat Med 2000;6:991–7.

47. Thannickal TC, Moore RY, Nienhuis R, et al. Reduced number of hypocretin neurons in human narcolepsy. Neuron 2000;27:469–74.

48. Hungs M, Lin L, Okun M, et al. Polymorphisms in the vicinity of the hypocretin/orexin are not associated with human narcolepsy. Neurology 2001;57:1893–5.

49. Olafsdottir BR, Rye DB, Scammell TE, et al. Polymorphisms in hypocretin/orexin pathway genes and narcolepsy. Neurology 2001;57:1896–9.

50. Miyagawa T, Honda M, Kawashima M, et al. Polymorphism located between CPT1B and CHKB, and HLA-DRB1*1501-DQB1*0602 haplotype confer susceptibility to CNS hypersomnias (essential hypersomnia). PLoS One 2009;4:e5394.

51. Hallmayer J, Faraco J, Lin L, et al. Narcolepsy is strongly associated with the T-cell receptor α locus. Nat Genet 2009;41:708–11.

52. Kalogiannis M, Grupke SL, Potter PE, et al. Narcoleptic orexin receptor knockout mice express enhanced cholinergic properties in laterodorsal tegmental neurons. Eur J Neurosci 2010;32:130–42.

53. Dauvilliers Y, Blouin JL, Neidhart E, et al. A narcolepsy susceptibility locus maps to a 5 Mb region of chromosome 21q. Ann Neurol 2004;56:382–8.

54. Nakayama J, Miura M, Honda M, et al. Linkage of human narcolepsy with HLA association to chromosome 4p13-q21. Genomics 2000;65:84–6.

55. Miyagawa T, Honda M, Kawashima M, et al. Polymorphism located in TCRA locus confers susceptibility to essential hypersomnia with HLA-DRB1*1501-DQB1*0602 haplotype. J Hum Genet 2010;55:63–5.

56. Padhan K, Varma R. Immunological synapse: a multi-protein signalling cellular apparatus for controlling gene expression. Immunology 2010;129:322–8.

57. Kornum BR, Kawashima M, Faraco J, et al. Common variants in P2RY11 are associated with narcolepsy. Nat Genet 2011;43:66–71.

58. Moore DJ, Chambers JK, Wahlin JP, et al. Expression pattern of human P2Y receptor subtypes: a quantitative reverse transcription-polymerase chain reaction study. Biochim Biophys Acta 2001; 1521:107–19.

59. Rosenbaum AI, Maxfield FR. Niemann-Pick type C disease: molecular mechanisms and potential therapeutic approaches. J Neurochem 2011;116: 789–95.

60. Vankova J, Stepanova I, Jech R, et al. Sleep disturbances and hypocretin deficiency in Niemann-Pick disease type C. Sleep 2003;26:427–30.

61. Vossler DG, Wyler AR, Wilkus RJ, et al. Cataplexy and monoamine oxidase deficiency in Norrie disease. Neurology 1996;46:1258–61.

62. Tobias ES, Tolmie JL, Stephenson JB. Cataplexy in the Prader-Willi syndrome. Arch Dis Child 2002;87:170.

63. Bruni O, Verrillo E, Novelli L, et al. Prader-Willi syndrome: sorting out the relationships between obesity, hypersomnia, and sleep apnea. Curr Opin Pulm Med 2010;16:568–73.

64. Mignot E, Lammers GJ, Ripley B, et al. The role of cerebrospinal fluid hypocretin measurement in the diagnosis of narcolepsy and other hypersomnias. Arch Neurol 2002;59:1553–62.

65. Melberg A, Hetta J, Dahl N, et al. Autosomal dominant cerebellar ataxia deafness and narcolepsy. J Neurol Sci 1995;134:119–29.

66. Melberg A, Dahl N, Hetta J, et al. Neuroimaging study in autosomal dominant cerebellar ataxia, deafness, and narcolepsy. Neurology 1999;53:2190–2.

67. Melberg A, Ripley B, Lin L, et al. Hypocretin deficiency in familial symptomatic narcolepsy. Ann Neurol 2001;49:136–7.

68. Stepien A, Staszewski J, Domzal TM, et al. Degenerative pontine lesions in patients with familial narcolepsy. Neurol Neurochir Pol 2010;44:21–7.

69. Arnulf I, Leu S, Oudiette D. Abnormal sleep and sleepiness in Parkinson's disease. Curr Opin Neurol 2008;21:472–7.

70. Lettre G, Rioux JD. Autoimmune diseases: insights from genome-wide association studies. Hum Mol Genet 2008;17:R116–21.

71. Kelley JM, Edberg JC, Kimberly RP. Pathways: strategies for susceptibility genes in SLE. Autoimmun Rev 2010;9:473–6.

72. Criswell LA. Gene discovery in rheumatoid arthritis highlights the CD40/NF-kappaB signaling pathway in disease pathogenesis. Immunol Rev 2010;233:55–61.

Genetics of Parasomnias

Thornton B.A. Mason II, MD, PhD, MSCE

KEYWORDS

• Parasomnias • Genetic factors • Disorders of arousal
• REM sleep

According to the *International Classification of Sleep Disorders*, second edition (ICSD-2), parasomnias are "undesirable physical events or experiences that occur during entry into sleep, within sleep, or during arousals from sleep."[1] The obvious, prolonged, dramatic events are most likely to raise concerns of patients, relatives, and clinicians, prompting medical evaluation.[2] As delineated by the ICSD-2, parasomnias are classified as: (1) disorders of arousal (from non–rapid eye movement, or NREM, sleep); (2) parasomnias usually associated with REM sleep; and (3) other parasomnias. While parasomnias are often believed to have multifactorial causes, there is growing support for significant genetic contributions to parasomnias. The goal of this review is to summarize the current understanding of genetic influences on parasomnias.

DISORDERS OF AROUSAL (FROM NREM SLEEP)

The disorders of arousal may be considered part of a continuum, as they share overlapping features: sleepwalking, confusional arousals, and sleep terrors. Although most often occurring in slow-wave sleep (stages 3 and 4 of NREM sleep), these parasomnias can also occur from stage 2 NREM sleep.[3] Common among these disorders include incomplete transition from slow-wave sleep, automatic behavior, altered perception of the environment, and variable degrees of amnesia for the event.[4] In particular, because of the association with slow-wave sleep, the arousal parasomnias tend to occur in the first third of the night, when slow-wave sleep is most prominent.[1] The sleep stage transition from slow-wave sleep is abnormal, often when shifting into lighter NREM sleep (eg, N2) just before the first REM sleep episode. The electroencephalograph (EEG) during these episodes demonstrates an admixture of theta, delta, and alpha frequencies.[5]

Multiple factors may influence arousal parasomnias. Age is an important issue, as many parasomnias are much more likely to occur in childhood rather than later in life. Another contributing factor includes the homeostatic drive to sleep, with more frequent or more severe parasomnia episodes being associated with prolonged sleep deprivation. Sleep deprivation has been shown to increase the complexity and frequency of sleepwalking events in a sleep laboratory during subsequent recovery nights; thus, sleep deprivation may facilitate a polysomnographically based diagnosis.[6] Other factors that may trigger parasomnias include medications (eg, neuroleptics, sedative hypnotics, stimulants, and antihistamines), a noisy or stimulating sleep environment, fever, stress, and intrinsic sleep disorders (such as obstructive sleep apnea and periodic limb movements in sleep).[7] There certainly are also familial patterns in the prevalence of parasomnias, supporting significant genetic factors.

There have been several approaches taken to assess genetic contributions to parasomnias. Motivation may be founded in the general observation that parasomnias are known to occur in families. Empirical family studies evaluate the prevalence of a parasomnia among relatives of an affected individual (proband); accordingly, the data indicate the presence of genetic effects, but do not prove genetic associations. Twin studies (monozygotic vs dizygotic) can be more helpful, with the assumption that environmental factors are equal for twins, and thus a greater similarity of monozygotic twins compared with dizygotic twins

Division of Neurology, The Children's Hospital of Philadelphia, 3501 Civic Center Boulevard, Philadelphia, PA 19104, USA
E-mail address: masont@email.chop.edu

Sleep Med Clin 6 (2011) 229–236
doi:10.1016/j.jsmc.2011.04.002

would support genetic factors.[8] Indeed, 3 different parameters can be modeled that could explain phenotypic variance: an additive genetic component; common or shared environmental components (physical environment, family, living conditions); and nonshared environmental components that affect a single twin (such as an illness or a hospitalization).[9]

Sleepwalking

Sleepwalking (somnambulism) may be either calm or agitated, with varying degrees of complexity and duration.[10] The frequency of sleepwalking may be underestimated because of episodes that are unobserved or unremembered.[11] In his landmark studies, Klackenberg[12] reported that the presence of sleepwalking of variable frequency was highest at 11 to 12 years, with males and females equally affected. Children with somnambulism are usually calm and do not demonstrate fear. The child may be found walking into a parent's room, bathroom, or different parts of the house. With mobility go concerns for safety, because patients with sleepwalking are at risk for injury. The patient may climb through windows, wander in bathrooms, attempt to walk downstairs, and sometimes leave the house. Injuries may include trauma from falls, lacerations from broken window/patio glass doors, and even hypothermia from exposure.[2]

Proposed modes of inheritance for sleepwalking include multifactorial models, autosomal recessive inheritance with incomplete penetrance, and autosomal dominant inheritance with variable penetrance.[13] Working from the Finnish Twin Cohort, Hublin and colleagues[11] reported that for sleepwalking in childhood the proband concordance rate was 0.55 for monozygotic and 0.35 for dizygotic pairs; in adults, the concordance rate was 0.32 for monozygotic and 0.06 for dizygotic pairs. Overall, the proportion of total phenotypic variance attributed to genetic influences was 57% in females and 66% in males in childhood sleepwalking, and 36% in women and 80% in men with adult sleepwalking. Lecendreux and colleagues,[13] in a family-based study, found a positive association between the HLA-DQB1*05 subtype and sleepwalking, suggesting a possible further interaction between the immune system and sleep.

A recent retrospective analysis of 7 families whose members had chronic sleepwalking demonstrated a complete overlap of sleepwalking and the presence of sleep-disordered breathing; moreover, individuals with ongoing sleepwalking who were treated for sleep-disordered breathing enjoyed improvement in sleepwalking episodes.[14]

It is unclear whether the chronic sleepwalking seen in these families resulted from inherited sleep cycle patterns that predisposed members to sleepwalking, or if prominent sleep-disordered breathing, from genetic factors, triggered sleepwalking episodes.

There has been a recent description of a 4-generation family with 9 individuals who sleepwalk and 13 unaffected.[15] Sleepwalking was inherited as an autosomal dominant trait with reduced penetrance. Linkage analysis revealed a genome-wide significant peak (logarithm of odds = 3.44) on chromosome 20q12-q13.12 between 55.6 and 61.4 cM.

Confusional Arousals

Confusional arousals have more associated agitation than what would be expected with sleepwalking. Confusional arousals occur mainly in infants and toddlers. A typical episode may begin with movements and moaning, then evolve to confused and agitated behavior with calling out, crying, or thrashing.[16] Attempts to wake the child fully are unsuccessful. The child appears confused, with eyes open or closed, and is very agitated or even combative. Physical injury is rarely seen.[17] A confusional arousal episode may last 5 to 15 minutes (although sometimes longer) before the child calms and returns to a restful sleep. In adults, sleep drunkenness (*schlaftrunkenheit*) can occur on rapid awakening from especially deep sleep. Factors that increase sleep drunkenness include sleep deprivation, medication effects, or other sleep disorders with excessive sleepiness or abnormal sleep/wake patterns.[2]

While genetic factors appear to play an important role,[8] detailed genetic studies on confusional arousals have not been performed. An increased frequency of confusional arousals and other arousal parasomnias (sleepwalking, sleep terrors) have been reported in both patients with nocturnal frontal lobe epilepsy and their relatives, as compared with controls; there may be a common underlying pathogenesis involving the cholinergic system and associated pathways. Understanding such associations might be furthered by evaluating families with the autosomal dominant form of frontal lobe epilepsy.[18]

Sleep Terrors

Sleep terrors are dramatic partial arousals from slow-wave sleep whereby the patient may sit up suddenly and scream, with an intense, blood-curdling "battle cry." The episode is a fight-flight phenomenon. Autonomic activation is present, with mydriasis, diaphoresis, and tachycardia.[19] There is increased respiratory tidal volume, and an intense look of fear on the face. Moreover, there is a "curious paradox" of endogenous arousal coexistent with external unarousability.[20] Sleep terrors are more prevalent in childhood than later life; peak prevalence is between 5 and 7 years, and resolution typically occurs before adolescence. Sleep terrors affect approximately 3% of children between the ages of 4 and 12 years and fewer than 1% of adults.[21]

There has long been evidence of a genetic risk factor for sleep terrors. Hällström[22] found support for inheritance in a 3-generation family, possibly consistent with an autosomal dominant disorder.[22] Kales and colleagues[23] reported that the prevalence of sleep terrors and sleepwalking in first-degree relatives of individuals with sleep terrors was 10 times greater than in the general population. These investigators estimated a 60% chance of a child being affected if both parents were affected. Ooki,[24] in a retrospective questionnaire-based study of junior high school monozygotic and dizygotic twins (881 pairs total), found that sleep terrors were under moderate to strong genetic control. In another Japanese study, Abe and colleagues[25] did not refer to "night terrors" in the questionnaire, but rather used a description they believed would be easily understood: "The child arises from fear and sits up in bed, does not recognize the mother or the surroundings, and cannot be awakened easily." Among 61 pairs of twins (47 monozygotic and 14 dizygotic), monozygotic twins were found to be significantly more concordant than dizygotic twins for night (sleep) terrors. Hublin and colleagues[26] performed a retrospective study using the adult Finnish twin population and found a higher polychoric correlation for childhood sleep terrors in monozygotic twins (0.38 for males; 0.35 females) than in dizygotic twins (0.17 males; 0.18 females).

In a large prospective study involving 390 pairs of monozygotic and dizygotic twins, Nguyen and colleagues[9] assessed the prevalence and frequency of sleep terrors at 18 months of age using a questionnaire administered to the biologic mother of the twins. Zygosity was established by questionnaire and genotyping, and for each type of twin the prevalence and polychoric correlation were calculated. Furthermore, the investigators used structural-equation modeling to determine the proportion of variance attributable to additive genetic, shared, and nonshared environmental factors. Among the results, affected children did not differ significantly by gender (51% girls, 49% boys). The polychoric correlation was calculated, which reflects the sleep terror tendency between the two members of each type of twin pair (monozygotic and dizygotic). Polychoric correlations were 0.63 for monozygotic and 0.36 for dizygotic twins at 18 months; at 30 months, they were 0.68 for monozygotic and 0.24 for dizygotic twins. Based on model-fitting analysis, there were significant genetic effects at 18 months that persisted as part of a 2-component model (43.7% additive genetic effects and 56.3% nonshared environment); at 30 months the model included 41.5% additive genetic effects and 58.5% nonshared environment.[9]

Nguyen and colleagues[9] caution that in their study (as well as in most other studies exploring genetic contributions to parasomnias) there was no objective laboratory evaluation to validate the questionnaire-based diagnosis. Sleep terrors were assessed by asking the biological mother the question: "Does your child have sleep terrors (this means sudden arousal with screams, sometimes with confusion and sweating)? Please circle one of the following answers: 1—never, 2—sometimes, 3—often, or 4—always." Some parents may have mistaken nightmares for sleep terrors, and vice versa. Also, sudden awakenings with crying may have been confused with sleep terrors.

It should be kept in mind, however, that a shared family environment complicates interpretation of heritability. Moreover, the heritability of sleep terrors could be secondary to other sleep disorders, as there is evidence of familial aggregation of restless legs syndrome[27–29] and sleep-disordered breathing.[30–32] Thus, other sleep disorders may result in familial sleep terrors indirectly.[33]

PARASOMNIAS USUALLY ASSOCIATED WITH REM SLEEP
REM Sleep Behavior Disorder

REM sleep behavior disorder (also known as REM sleep motor disorder) involves "problematic behavioral release," with enacting of unpleasant, combative dreams. Rather than manifesting the expected REM sleep atonia, patients with REM sleep behavior disorder have complex movements that can be vigorous and even violent. Thus affected patients, while in a dream state, may injure themselves or their bed partners by punching, grabbing, or kicking.[17,34] As a result, trauma can occur (eg, lacerations, ecchymoses, and fractures) that may be at times severe and perhaps life-threatening. Patients with REM sleep behavior disorder report that their dreams have more action, intensity, and violence than typical dreams.[35] While there is variable loss of the general muscle paralysis typically associated with REM sleep, all other major features of REM sleep remain intact in REM sleep behavior disorder. Other aspects of generalized anomalous motor control in REM sleep behavior disorder include periodic limb movements and nonperiodic limb twitching in NREM sleep.

REM sleep behavior disorder tends to have a male predominance, with onset usually in the sixth to seventh decade of life; in a major case series, 25% of patients experienced a prodrome with a mean duration of 22 years (range 2–48 years), where vocalizations and partial limb movements without complex behavior occurred during REM sleep. REM sleep behavior disorder has been found in multiple neurodegenerative disorders.[1] Accordingly, there are reports, for example, of specific gene mutations for parkinsonism (parkin) and Machado-Joseph disease (SCA-3) associated with REM sleep behavior disorder.[36,37]

Recurrent Isolated Sleep Paralysis

Sleep paralysis is a generalized, fleeting inability to speak or to move the trunk, head, and limbs that occurs during the transitional period between sleep and wakefulness. The episodes last variably from 1 minute or less to several minutes.[38] There is preservation of consciousness. Despite their relative brevity, episodes of sleep paralysis can be quite distressing, especially if associated with hallucinations.[38] The sleep paralysis phenomenon is known in many cultures, and has been named "Old Hag" in Newfoundland, "Kokma" in the West Indies, "Kanashibari" in Japan, and "being ridden by the witch" by some southern United States African Americans.[39] Sleep paralysis may occur as part of the classic tetrad of narcolepsy, as an isolated form in otherwise healthy individuals, or in a familial form apparently under genetic control.[40] Factors such as fatigue, stress, irregular schedules, shift work, sleeping in a supine position, alcohol/caffeine use, and sleep deprivation may predispose individuals to sleep paralysis.[38,40] Mental disorders associated with sleep paralysis include panic disorder, other anxiety disorders, bipolar disorder, posttraumatic stress disorder, and depression.[39] Few reports exist that explore possible genetic factors in sleep paralysis[1]; one study of 22 patients with sleep paralysis found a positive family history of sleep paralysis in 19 (86%).[41] Two families have been reported with apparent familial sleep paralysis present over 3 and 4 generations; a maternal form of transmission has been suggested.[1]

OTHER PARASOMNIAS
Enuresis

Nocturnal enuresis (bedwetting) refers to the passing of urine while asleep. In young children,

less than 5 years of age, nocturnal enuresis is normal. It has been estimated that at 5 years approximately 15% to 25% of children have nocturnal enuresis.[42] The prevalence of nocturnal enuresis is approximately 1.5 to 2 times greater in boys than girls.[43] With each advancing year, the percentage of children with nocturnal enuresis decreases by about 15%[42,44,45]; this steady decrease may reflect interim maturation of central nervous system voiding mechanisms or the bladder.[46] In adolescence, only 1% to 3% are found to still wet the bed.

Enuresis can be classified according to time of day (nocturnal enuresis, diurnal enuresis), periods of dryness, and the presence of other symptoms. Primary enuresis refers to enuresis in a child with who has never been dry (continent) consistently since birth, whereas secondary enuresis is applicable to a child who has had at least 6 months of dryness before recurrence of enuresis. Another terminology applies to conditions where there may be other symptoms or complications associated with the child's enuresis. Monosymptomatic or uncomplicated nocturnal enuresis involves normal voiding at night in bed without other symptoms referable to the urogenital or gastrointestinal tracts. On the other hand, polysymptomatic (or complicated) nocturnal enuresis refers to bedwetting that is associated with daytime symptoms, such as severe urgency, staccato voiding (inappropriate voluntary control of the external urinary sphincter), urge incontinence (inability to inhibit a bladder contraction and/or inadequate bladder capacity), chronic constipation, or encopresis.[42,44]

Genetic and familial factors may play a role in enuresis. From a family history perspective, enuresis is increased in the offspring of parents who had childhood enuresis. It has been reported, for example, that if both parents have a history of enuresis there is a 77% risk of their children also developing enuresis. With only a single parent having been enuretic, the risk decreases to 43%. In cases where neither parent had enuresis during childhood, a much lower risk for affected children has been reported (15%).[47] Abe and colleagues[25] evaluated enuresis among 72 monozygotic and 21 dizygotic twin pairs at 3 years of age, and found that nocturnal enuresis was significantly more concordant among monozygotic than dizygotic twins. Segregation analysis in enuresis points to a complex pattern of inheritance.[48] Autosomal dominant inheritance with high penetrance, followed by autosomal dominant inheritance with low penetrance and an autosomal recessive mode, has been described.[8] Eiberg and colleagues,[48] for example, identified 11 families with primary enuresis that appeared to follow an autosomal dominant mode of inheritance with a penetrance exceeding 90%; the investigators found strong evidence of linkage on chromosome 13q13-q14.2. In a subsequent study, Arnell and colleagues[49] evaluated genetic factors and the pattern of inheritance for primary nocturnal enuresis in 392 families. In 43%, dominant transmission was observed, whereas an apparent recessive inheritance was observed in 9% of the families; the majority of probands were males, by a ratio of 3:1. Linkage studies supported a possible gene locus on chromosome 12q being associated with nocturnal enuresis. More recently, a preliminary study explored endothelial and nitric oxide synthase (NOS) gene polymorphisms in children with primary nocturnal enuresis; the findings suggested that a neuronal NOS gene polymorphism may be associated with nocturnal enuresis in a subset of children, although further studies with larger sample sizes are needed to evaluate this finding.[50]

Sleep-Related Dissociative Disorders

Dissociative disorders involve a disruption of the usually integrated functions of consciousness, memory, identity, or perception of the environment. The 3 categories of dissociative disorders that have been documented with respect to sleep-related dissociative disorders include dissociative fugue (a disturbed state of consciousness whereby a patient appears fully aware in performing activities but subsequently has no recollection), dissociative identity disorder (formerly called multiple personality disorder), and dissociative disorder not otherwise specified. Most patients with sleep-related dissociative disorders have corresponding daytime dissociative disorders, and a current or previous history of physical or sexual abuse.[1] Childhood traumatic events may result in the development of dissociative symptoms, possibly serving as a defense mechanism. There appears to be an association between nightmares and dissociative states or experiences. Agargun and colleagues,[51] for example, found a strong association in college students between nightmares and childhood traumatic experiences. Patients with dissociative disorders also often experience nightmare disorder; those patients with dissociative disorders and nightmare disorder have been reported to have a higher rate of suicide attempts, self-mutilatory behavior, and comorbidity with borderline personality disorder than those without nightmare disorder.[52] During the sleep-related behaviors, patients can run, scream, or display sexualized behavior. These activities may represent reenactment of previous abusive situations;

there is amnesia for the behavior on the following day. The age of onset can range from childhood to middle adulthood.

There are reports of apparent familial clustering of dissociative disorders, which in turn raises the issue of the relative roles of environmental factors as compared with genetic contributions. Twin studies have been used in attempts to sort out phenotypic variance due to shared environment (ie, environmental influences that produce sibling similarity in dissociation), nonshared environment (resulting in sibling differentiation), or genetics (in monozygotic and dizygotic twins). Waller and Ross,[53] in a study of adolescent twins, reported that variance in dissociation was caused by combinations of environmental factors but not by genetics. On the other hand, Jang and colleagues,[54] in their study of adult twins, describe very different results, with 48% of the variance in their twin sample being due to additive genetic influences. More recently, Becker-Blease and colleagues[55] examined child and adolescent twins, and also found that hereditability was significant at 59%, with the balance of the variance attributed to the nonshared environmental component.

Two studies have implicated specific genetic polymorphisms in the clinical expression of dissociation. Koenen and colleagues[56] explored polymorphisms in FKBP5, which encodes a glucocorticoid receptor–regulating co-chaperone of stress proteins. Two single nucleotide polymorphisms were significantly associated with peritraumatic dissociation in medically injured children (eg, from motor vehicle accidents, physical assaults, and falls). This significance persisted after controlling for sex, age, race, and injury severity, and the proportion of the variance in dissociation explained by the polymorphisms ranged from 14% to 27%.[56] Savitz and colleagues[57] evaluated the interaction of a catechol-O-methyltransferase polymorphism (Val158Met) on perceived dissociation, and found that the Val/Val genotype was associated with increasing levels of dissociation in the setting of higher childhood trauma, whereas the reverse was true for the Met/Met genotype (that was essentially protective from dissociation). These intriguing findings clearly need to be replicated in other sample populations before their general significance can be evaluated.

Exploding Head Syndrome

Exploding head syndrome (EHS) is a harmless but potentially terrifying situation that usually occurs while a patient is falling asleep, but occasionally may occur on awakening. Patients report a terrifying loud noise, sometimes accompanied by the perception of a flash of light or myoclonic jerks. The episode lasts only an instant; afterwards, the patient may experience palpitations and acute anxiety.[58] In most cases, EHS is not associated with sudden pain or headache.[59,60] Polysomnography has verified that EHS attacks occur during wakefulness rather than bona fide sleep; the attacks are not associated with pathologic or epileptiform EEG changes.[60] Onset of EHS episodes may occur during childhood, but most commonly begin in middle age or later.[58] Attacks are variable, and may be sporadic; periods when EHS episodes recur may be related to stressful situations at school, work, or home.[60] Although occasional cases of EHS may occur in the same family, it is unclear if true familial patterns exist.[1]

Sleep-Related Eating Disorder

Sleep-related eating disorder has combined characteristics of sleepwalking and daytime eating disorders (such as the compulsive eating of binge-eating disorder or bulimia nervosa). Patients with sleep-related eating disorder experience a partial arousal from sleep, often 2 to 3 hours after sleep onset. Their subsequent eating is "out of control" (rapid and sloppy, often with high carbohydrate foods, and sometimes taken in bizarre combinations of food items that may include nonnutritive substances). Patients may become agitated or angry if they are disturbed during an episode, and have limited to no recall of the episode the following day.[61] Common responses to nocturnal eating include morning anorexia or restriction of daytime eating. In a case series of 23 patients with sleep-related eating disorder, Winkelman[61] reported that 3 had onset before age 10 years, with the majority having onset in adolescence or early adulthood. Medications that increase the risk of sleep-related eating disorder include triazolam abuse, olanzapine, and respiridone.[62,63] In addition to sleep-related eating disorder, the differential diagnosis of nocturnal eating includes the following: nocturnal eating syndrome (eating at night with full alertness), binge-eating disorder or bulimia nervosa with nocturnal eating (eating at night with full alertness, combined with a daytime eating disorder), dissociative disorder with nocturnal eating (eating at night and altered level of awareness in the setting of disorders such as multiple personality disorder, posttraumatic stress disorder), and Kleine-Levin syndrome.[61] Although genetic factors would seem plausible given the overlap with sleepwalking, no detailed family studies for sleep-related eating disorder have been conducted to date.

Catathrenia

Catathrenia, or nocturnal groaning, can occur in NREM sleep (stage 2) and REM sleep.[64] The moaning/groaning sounds are in expiration only, and last 2 to 20 seconds; the sounds tend to be repeated in clusters of a few minutes to an hour, and occur several times nightly. Polysomnography has shown that catathrenia is associated with a slightly decreased heart rate and moderately positive intraesophageal pressure. The groaning terminates with a snort, followed by rebound in heart rate. The onset of catathrenia may begin during childhood or adolescence.[64] The etiology of this groaning is unclear, as no underlying psychiatric or respiratory disease has been found. Although catathrenia may have an adverse social impact, no specific therapy has been found to be effective. Moreover, no definite family pattern or specific genetic contributors have been reported.

SUMMARY

The parasomnias are fascinating disorders that show dynamic relationships with patient age, sleep debt, environmental factors, and even psychopathology. In some cases, such as the arousal parasomnias, familial patterns are well established; in other disorders, such as catathrenia and EHS, convincing family studies are lacking. Given the challenging clinical variability of parasomnias, future studies require more careful phenotyping of cases as well as finer scrutiny of noninherited contributory factors and other concurrent sleep pathology. The potential benefits of such investigations could be large, in terms of not only an enhanced understanding of these particular sleep disorders but also a greater knowledge of arousal mechanisms and sleep/wake transitions across the general population.

REFERENCES

1. AASM. International classification of sleep disorders: diagnostic and coding manual. 2nd edition. Westchester (IL): American Academy of Sleep Medicine; 2005.
2. Stores G. Dramatic parasomnias. J R Soc Med 2001;94:173–6.
3. Broughton R. NREM arousal parasomnias. In: Kryger MH R, Roth T, Dement WC, editors. Principles and practice of sleep medicine. 3rd edition. Philadelphia: W.B. Saunders Co.; 2000. p. 693–706.
4. Mason TB 2nd, Pack AI. Pediatric parasomnias. Sleep 2007;30:141–51.

5. Mahowald MW, Ettinger MG. Things that go bump in the night: the parasomnias revisited. J Clin Neurophysiol 1990;7:119–43.

6. Joncas S, Zadra A, Paquet J, et al. The value of sleep deprivation as a diagnostic tool in adult sleepwalkers. Neurology 2002;58:936–40.

7. Mahowald MW, Schenck CH, Rosen GM, et al. The role of a sleep disorder center in evaluating sleep violence. Arch Neurol 1992;49:604–7.

8. Hublin C, Kaprio J. Genetic aspects and genetic epidemiology of parasomnias. Sleep Med Rev 2003;7:413–21.

9. Nguyen BH, Perusse D, Paquet J, et al. Sleep terrors in children: a prospective study of twins. Pediatrics 2008;122:e1164–7.

10. Mahowald MW, Bornemann MC, Schenck CH. Parasomnias. Semin Neurol 2004;24:283–92.

11. Hublin C, Kaprio J, Partinen M, et al. Prevalence and genetics of sleepwalking: a population-based twin study. Neurology 1997;48:177–81.

12. Klackenberg G. Somnambulism in childhood—prevalence, course and behavioral correlations. A prospective longitudinal study (6–16 years). Acta Paediatr Scand 1982;71:495–9.

13. Lecendreux M, Bassetti C, Dauvilliers Y, et al. HLA and genetic susceptibility to sleepwalking. Mol Psychiatry 2003;8:114–7.

14. Cao M, Guilleminault C. Families with sleepwalking. Sleep Med 2010;11:726–34.

15. Licis AK, Desruisseau DM, Yamada KA, et al. Novel genetic findings in an extended family pedigree with sleepwalking. Neurology 2011;76:49–52.

16. Rosen GM, Ferber R, Mahowald MW. Evaluation of parasomnias in children. Child Adolesc Psychiatr Clin N Am 1996;5:601–16.

17. Sheldon SH. Parasomnias in childhood. Pediatr Clin North Am 2004;51:69–88, vi.

18. Bisulli F, Vignatelli L, Naldi I, et al. Increased frequency of arousal parasomnias in families with nocturnal frontal lobe epilepsy: a common mechanism? Epilepsia 2010;51:1852–60.

19. Mason TB 2nd, Pack AI. Sleep terrors in childhood. J Pediatr 2005;147:388–92.

20. Mahowald M. Arousal and sleep-wake transition parasomnias. In: Lee-Chiong TL, Sateia MJ, Carskadon MA, editors. Sleep medicine. Philadelphia: Hanley and Belfus, Inc; 2002. p. 207–13.

21. Robinson A, Guilleminault C. Disorders of arousal. In: Chokroverty S, Hening W, Walters AS, editors. Sleep and movement disorders. Philadelphia: Butterworth Heinemann; 2003. p. 265–72.

22. Hällström T. Night terror in adults through three generations. Acta Psychiatr Scand 1972;48:350–2.

23. Kales A, Soldatos CR, Bixler EO, et al. Hereditary factors in sleepwalking and night terrors. Br J Psychiatry 1980;137:111–8.

24. Ooki S. Statistical genetic analysis of some problem behaviors during sleep in childhood—estimation of genetic and environmental factors influencing multiple health phenomena simultaneously. Nippon Eiseigaku Zasshi 2000;55:489–99.

25. Abe K, Oda N, Ikenaga K, et al. Twin study on night terrors, fears, and some physiological and behavioural characteristics in childhood. Psychiatr Genet 1993;3:39–43.

26. Hublin C, Kaprio J, Partinen M, et al. Limits of self-report in assessing sleep terrors in a population survey. Sleep 1999;22:89–93.

27. Desautels A, Turecki G, Montplaisir J, et al. Identification of a major susceptibility locus for restless legs syndrome on chromosome 12q. Am J Hum Genet 2001;69:1266–70.

28. Winkelmann J, Muller-Myhsok B, Wittchen HU, et al. Complex segregation analysis of restless legs syndrome provides evidence for an autosomal dominant mode of inheritance in early age at onset families. Ann Neurol 2002;52:297–302.

29. Bonati MT, Ferini-Strambi L, Aridon P, et al. Autosomal dominant restless legs syndrome maps on chromosome 14q. Brain 2003;126:1485–92.

30. Redline S, Tishler PV, Schluchter M, et al. Risk factors for sleep-disordered breathing in children. Associations with obesity, race, and respiratory problems. Am J Respir Crit Care Med 1999;159:1527–32.

31. Morton S, Rosen C, Larkin E, et al. Predictors of sleep-disordered breathing in children with a history of tonsillectomy and/or adenoidectomy. Sleep 2001;24:823–9.

32. Buxbaum SG, Elston RC, Tishler PV, et al. Genetics of the apnea hypopnea index in Caucasians and African Americans: I. Segregation analysis. Genet Epidemiol 2002;22:243–53.

33. Guilleminault C, Palombini L, Pelayo R, et al. Sleepwalking and sleep terrors in prepubertal children: what triggers them? Pediatrics 2003;111:e17–25.

34. Schenck CH, Bundlie SR, Ettinger MG, et al. Chronic behavioral disorders of human REM sleep: a new category of parasomnia. Sleep 1986;9:293–308.

35. Schenck CH, Mahowald MW. REM sleep behavior disorder: clinical, developmental, and neuroscience perspectives 16 years after its formal identification in SLEEP. Sleep 2002;25:120–38.

36. Kumru H, Santamaria J, Tolosa E, et al. Rapid eye movement sleep behavior disorder in parkinsonism with parkin mutations. Ann Neurol 2004;56:599–603.

37. Rye DB, Johnston LH, Watts RL, et al. Juvenile Parkinson's disease with REM sleep behavior disorder, sleepiness, and daytime REM onset. Neurology 1999;53:1868–70.

38. Ohayon MM, Zulley J, Guilleminault C, et al. Prevalence and pathologic associations of sleep

paralysis in the general population. Neurology 1999;52:1194–200.

39. Paradis CM, Friedman S. Sleep paralysis in African Americans with panic disorder. Transcult Psychiatry 2005;42:123–34.

40. Buzzi G, Cirignotta F. Isolated sleep paralysis: a web survey. Sleep Res Online 2000;3:61–6.

41. Dahlitz M, Parkes JD. Sleep paralysis. Lancet 1993; 341:406–7.

42. Thiedke CC. Nocturnal enuresis. Am Fam Physician 2003;67:1499–506.

43. Kajiwara M, Inoue K, Kato M, et al. Nocturnal enuresis and overactive bladder in children: an epidemiological study. Int J Urol 2006;13:36–41.

44. Tietjen DN, Husmann DA. Nocturnal enuresis: a guide to evaluation and treatment. Mayo Clin Proc 1996;71:857–62.

45. Laberge L, Tremblay RE, Vitaro F, et al. Development of parasomnias from childhood to early adolescence. Pediatrics 2000;106:67–74.

46. Weissbach A, Leiberman A, Tarasiuk A, et al. Adenotonsillectomy improves enuresis in children with obstructive sleep apnea syndrome. Int J Pediatr Otorhinolaryngol 2006;70:1351–6.

47. Norgaard JP, Djurhuus JC, Watanabe H, et al. Experience and current status of research into the pathophysiology of nocturnal enuresis. Br J Urol 1997;79:825–35.

48. Eiberg H, Berendt I, Mohr J. Assignment of dominant inherited nocturnal enuresis (ENUR1) to chromosome 13q. Nat Genet 1995;10:354–6.

49. Arnell H, Hjalmas K, Jagervall M, et al. The genetics of primary nocturnal enuresis: inheritance and suggestion of a second major gene on chromosome 12q. J Med Genet 1997;34:360–5.

50. Balat A, Alasehirli B, Oguzkan S, et al. Nitric oxide synthase gene polymorphisms in children with primary nocturnal enuresis: a preliminary study. Ren Fail 2007;29:79–83.

51. Agargun MY, Kara H, Ozer OA, et al. Nightmares and dissociative experiences: the key role of childhood traumatic events. Psychiatry Clin Neurosci 2003;57:139–45.

52. Agargun MY, Kara H, Ozer OA, et al. Clinical importance of nightmare disorder in patients with dissociative disorders. Psychiatry Clin Neurosci 2003;57:575–9.

53. Waller NG, Ross C. The prevalence and biometric structure of pathological dissociation in the general population: taxometric and behavior genetic findings. J Abnorm Psychol 1997;106:499–510.

54. Jang KL, Paris J, Zweig-Frank H, et al. Twin study of dissociative experience. J Nerv Ment Dis 1998;186:345–51.

55. Becker-Blease K, Deater-Deckard K, Eley, et al. A genetic analysis of individual differences in dissociative behaviors in childhood and adolescence. J Child Psychol Psychiatry 2004;45:522–32.

56. Koenen KC, Saxe G, Purcell S, et al. Polymorphisms in FKBP5 are associated with peritraumatic dissociation in medically injured children. Mol Psychiatry 2005;10:1058–9.

57. Savitz J, van der Merwe L, Newman T, et al. The relationship between child abuse and dissociation: is it influenced by catechol-O-methyltransferase (COMT) activity? Int J Neuropsychopharmacol 2008;11:149–61.

58. Evans RW, Pearce JM. Exploding head syndrome. Headache 2001;41:602–3.

59. Jacome DE. Exploding head syndrome and idiopathic stabbing headache relieved by nifedipine. Cephalalgia 2001;21:617–8.

60. Sachs C, Svanborg E. The exploding head syndrome: polysomnographic recordings and therapeutic suggestions. Sleep 1991;14:263–6.

61. Winkelman JW. Clinical and polysomnographic features of sleep-related eating disorder. J Clin Psychiatry 1998;59:14–9.

62. Lu ML, Shen WW. Sleep-related eating disorder induced by risperidone. J Clin Psychiatry 2004;65:273–4.

63. Paquet V, Strul J, Servais L, et al. Sleep-related eating disorder induced by olanzapine. J Clin Psychiatry 2002;63:597.

64. Vetrugno R, Provini F, Plazzi G, et al. Catathrenia (nocturnal groaning): a new type of parasomnia. Neurology 2001;56:681–3.

Genetics of Sleep Apnea

Allan I. Pack, MBChB, PhD

KEYWORDS

• Obstructive sleep apnea • Genetics • Obesity • Replication

Obstructive sleep apnea (OSA) is a common disorder with multiple adverse consequences.[1–3] This disorder leads to excessive sleepiness, with increased risk of motor vehicle crashes,[1] and is an independent risk factor for cardiovascular disease[2] and insulin resistance.[3] However, not all patients with OSA get all these consequences. There is a differential susceptibility to these consequences. Even patients with severe OSA may not complain of excessive sleepiness. It is likely that this differential susceptibility is in part genetic, which complicates identifying genes conferring risk for OSA because patients with consequences, such as excessive sleepiness, are more likely to present clinically. In this article, the evidence that there is a genetic contribution to OSA is reviewed. The likely intermediate traits are discussed, each of which may have genetic contributions. The studies identifying gene variants conferring risk for OSA are described. The studies of the genetic determinants of cardiovascular consequences of OSA are also described in the contribution by Ryan and colleagues in this issue. At present, there are no firmly established gene variants conferring risk for OSA, which have been replicated in several studies. In all genetic studies, replication is the key and adds confidence to the findings.[4]

FAMILIAL AGGREGATION OF OSA

The original demonstration that OSA may have a familial basis came from the study of a single family with a high prevalence of OSA.[5] This observation led to studies to first address familial aggregation of the symptoms for OSA, such as habitual snoring and excessive sleepiness, snorting, gasping, and apneas. These symptoms aggregate in families.[6] This assessment was followed by studies assessing apneas and hypopneas during sleep that were conducted in the United States,[7,8] Israel,[9] Scotland,[10] and Iceland.[11]

Familial aggregation was shown in the Cleveland Family Study.[7] This study is important and, as described later, has been the basis of many genetic investigations of OSA. The design of this study is described. In this study, probands with OSA were identified (n = 230) who had an apnea-hypopnea index (AHI) greater than 20 events per hour or were considered to have severe-enough OSA to warrant therapy. Family members, including first-degree relatives, selected second-degree relatives, and spouses, had overnight sleep studies largely using equipment that did not include electroencephalographic assessment of sleep. Neighborhood controls and their relatives were also studied using the same strategy. There was an increased relative risk of OSA in first-degree relatives of probands with OSA, which was not affected by controlling for body mass index (BMI, calculated as the weight in kilograms divided by the height in meters squared) as a covariate. Thus, this familial aggregation of OSA cannot simply be explained by obesity. Obesity is the major risk factor for OSA in middle-aged adults,[12] and it too is heritable.[13–16]

That obesity is not sufficient to explain the familial aggregation of OSA is further supported by findings from the study by Mathur and Douglas[10] from Scotland. In this study, the prevalence of OSA in first-degree relatives of less-obese individuals with OSA (BMI<30 kg/m^2) was compared with that in controls chosen at random from a list of patients in a primary care practice. Controls were matched for age, gender, height, and weight. First-degree relatives had higher levels of sleep-disordered breathing than controls. In particular, first-degree

Division of Sleep Medicine, Department of Medicine, Center for Sleep and Circadian Neurobiology, Translational Research Laboratories, University of Pennsylvania School of Medicine, 125 South 31st Street, Suite 2100, Philadelphia, PA 19104-3403, USA
E-mail address: pack@mail.med.upenn.edu

Sleep Med Clin 6 (2011) 237–245
doi:10.1016/j.jsmc.2011.04.007
1556-407X/11/$ – see front matter © 2011 Elsevier Inc. All rights reserved.

relatives of patients had more-frequent moderate OSA (AHI>15 events per hour) and severe OSA (AHI>30 events per hour) than controls. All individuals in this study had a cephalometric analysis performed. This analysis revealed that first-degree relatives of patients with OSA had more retroposed mandibles and maxillae than controls. Thus, part of the increased OSA in first-degree relatives of patients is likely related to the craniofacial risk factors for OSA that are described more fully later. These differences in craniofacial structure, although significant, are relatively subtle. There were also differences in airway size between relatives of probands and controls. The airway was smaller in the relatives of probands than in controls.

The study in Iceland used a different approach[11]—a genealogy strategy—that is relatively unique to Iceland. This small island, with a population of about 300,000, was settled between 900 and 1100 AD. There was little subsequent emigration to Iceland. Icelanders are wonderful record keepers. deCODE Genetics took advantage of this record keeping and used birth and marriage records to create the genealogy of the country going back over centuries. This compilation allowed family relationships of cases with a particular disorder to be defined in a database and allowed the examination of individuals with different degrees of relatedness. In Iceland, there is also an active program for the diagnosis and treatment of OSA that is provided by the single-payer health care system. All patients in Iceland who are identified to have OSA are referred to the main University Hospital in Reykjavik to start nasal continuous positive airway pressure. When all cases of patients with OSA diagnosed between 1979 and 1999 were examined, it was found that these patients were more related then randomly selected controls, that is, there was a significantly higher kinship coefficient.[11] First-degree relatives of patients with OSA had an approximately 2-fold increased risk of OSA.[11] It is possible that this increased risk of OSA in relatives in this study is related to them being more likely to seek clinical evaluation for OSA as a result of knowledge gained from their relatives. However, diagnosis of OSA in Iceland is approaching population estimates of prevalence.

For review of these early studies of genetics of sleep apnea, the readers are referred to the article by Redline and Tishler.[17]

SEGREGATION ANALYSES

In the Cleveland Family Study, models were used to assess the likely pattern of inheritance of OSA.[18] The data from whites of European origin and African Americans were analyzed separately, and these modeling studies suggested a different mode of inheritance in the two ethnicities.[18] Whites showed a pattern of inheritance that suggested a recessive mode of inheritance with a single major gene.[18] The inheritance pattern was attenuated when BMI was introduced into the models. In contrast, in African Americans, adjusting for BMI actually increased the evidence for segregation of a codominant gene.[18] That different patterns of inheritance seem to be the basis of OSA in these two ethnic groups has led all subsequent investigations in the Cleveland Family Study doing studies separately in each ethnic group.

INTERMEDIATE TRAITS FOR SLEEP APNEA

There are several intermediate traits for OSA. Obesity is an important risk factor for OSA[12] and is heritable.[13–16] Other intermediate traits are structural, involving craniofacial structure and size of relevant upper airway soft tissue structures. Other traits involved include neural control of the upper airway, and it has been proposed that metabolic and other pathways may also be involved.[17]

Obesity

An important pathway to OSA is obesity. Obesity is a strong risk factor for OSA[12]; this is particularly true in middle-aged adults. In the elderly, the association between OSA and obesity is less.[19,20] Studying the genetics of OSA in the elderly may therefore be of value to identify nonobesity gene variants because in younger individuals, the obesity pathway is quite major. It is useful conceptually to consider obesity and nonobesity genetic pathways for OSA.[21]

Although obesity is a major risk factor for OSA, the mechanism is unknown. One recently identified possibility is fat being directly deposited in the tongue, increasing tongue size and compromising airway size. This concept originally came from autopsy studies in humans.[22] There are distinct areas of fat deposition in the tongue, and the amount of fat in the tongue is strongly associated with the BMI. In this study, it is unknown if subjects had OSA or not. This study in humans is supported by findings in a mouse model of obesity. The New Zealand obese (NZO) mouse sleeps upright, suggesting that it may have upper airway compromise.[23] (The NZO mouse is derived by a polygenetic mutation on the New Zealand wild-type background.) Magnetic resonance imaging studies show that the NZO mouse has a larger tongue than lean controls.[23] Histologic studies reveal fat deposits between muscle fibers in the tongue. The upper airway of the NZO mouse is also smaller than that of wild-type controls.[23] Thus, the relationship between obesity and OSA may be explained by a particular type of fat distribution, that is, fat deposits in the tongue.

Obesity is typically assessed by the BMI. BMI is a heritable trait, with estimates of heritability of the order of 40%.[13-16] There have been several genome-wide association studies (GWAS) examining association with obesity both as a dichotomous trait, for example, overweight BMI greater than 27.5 kg/m^2 or obese BMI greater than 30.0 kg/m^2, and with BMI as a continuous variable. There has been a recent meta-analysis of these studies that looked for association with around 2.8 million single nucleotide polymorphisms (SNPs) in up to 123,865 individuals, with a targeted follow-up of 42 SNPs identified in the first phase of the analysis in 125,931 additional individuals.[24] This study is massive and indicates the type of sample sizes needed when the trait of interest is polygenetic (as is likely the case for OSA), with each gene variant conferring a modest effect. The meta-analysis confirmed 14 known obesity susceptibility genes and identified 18 new loci (see list in original publication). The gene variant that showed the most significant association with obesity and accounted for the most variance (albeit very small) was in the fat mass and obesity (FTO) gene. Recently, much has been learned about the biology of the FTO gene.[25] The FTO gene is widely expressed but is most highly expressed in the hypothalamus. Expression of the FTO gene in the arcuate nucleus of the hypothalamus, an area involved in feeding control, is increased when mice are fed a high-fat diet[26] and decreased with fasting.[27] Changing expression of the FTO gene in this brain region also alters feeding. Specifically, increasing expression of the FTO gene in the arcuate nucleus of the hypothalamus in mice reduces food intake, whereas knocking down expression with RNA interference increases food intake.[26] This is an example of how findings from GWAS and human genetic studies can lead to identifying the function of an entirely new biological pathway.[25]

Although much is known, therefore, about the genes conferring risk of obesity, much remains to be discovered. The 32 variants identified explain only 1.45% of the variance in BMI and only 2% to 4% of estimated heritability.[24] At present, it is not known whether these gene variants are part of the obesity pathway to OSA as seems likely. This role needs to be assessed as does whether there are gene variants that play a role in determining fat deposition in the tongue.

Craniofacial Structure

Early cephalometric studies showed differences in craniofacial structure between patients with OSA

and age- and gender-matched controls.[28,29] These differences are most marked in those with nonobese sleep apnea.[30] Although several differences have been demonstrated in patients with OSA, meta-analyses indicate that the most robust finding is a reduced mandibular length in patients with OSA.[28] The role of reduced mandibular length has also been shown in a recent study in Japanese men.[31] The relative role of craniofacial changes, soft tissue changes, and obesity is different between ethnic groups.[32] Comparing whites in Australia with Asians in Hong Kong with similar degrees of OSA, the Asians had a reduced craniofacial base and mandibular length, that is, craniofacial risk factors played a larger role in this group. In contrast, the whites were more obese and had larger tongue volumes, that is, soft tissue risk factors played a larger role. There are also differences in craniofacial features between African Americans with OSA and whites with OSA.[33] Brachycephaly is associated with OSA in whites but not in African Americans.

Heritability of these craniofacial structural risk factors has been demonstrated in several studies. In general, twin studies of craniofacial structure by cephalometric analyses show high heritability of craniofacial dimensions.[34,35] With respect to OSA, specifically the study in Edinburgh, Scotland mentioned earlier[10] showed that first-degree relatives of probands with OSA had, as compared with controls, more retroposition of the maxilla and mandible and longer soft palates. In a study by Guilleminault and colleagues[8] in California, relatives of patients with OSA had more retroposed mandibles and more inferiorly placed hyoid bones. Inferior position of the hyoid bone in patients with OSA has been demonstrated in several studies.[36-38] But recent data suggest that this inferior position of the hyoid bone is not a primary risk factor but rather is secondary to the increased tongue volume in patients with OSA.[39] Specifically, the differences in hyoid bone position between patients with OSA and controls are no longer present when tongue volume is introduced into the analysis as a covariate.

Thus, the key craniofacial variables that are risk factors for OSA, which are heritable, are retroposed mandible and reduced mandibular length. Although these variables are relatively simple to measure in a large number of subjects, at present, there are no studies analyzing the genetics of this aspect of the phenotype. New approaches involving analysis of digital photographs of the face are promising in this regard.[40]

Soft Tissue Structures

There is also familial aggregation of the volume of upper airway structures that are risk factors for

OSA.[41] Studies of probands with OSA, and their first-degree same-gender relatives, as well as age- and gender-matched controls, and their same-gender first-degree relatives, show small differences within families but large differences between families, that is, patients and controls, as well as between first-degree relatives of patients and controls. These differences result in moderate heritability[41] for volumes of key structures that have been shown to be associated with increased risk for OSA.[42] In particular, the heritability for volume of the lateral pharyngeal walls is 25.6%, for tongue volume 37.8%, and for volume of total soft tissues in the upper airway 41.3%. This study did not assess fat deposition in the tongue or other upper airway structures. But fat deposition seems an unlikely explanation for this heritability because after adjusting for age, gender, craniofacial size, race, and total neck fat volume, heritability estimates either increase (lateral wall volume from 25.6%–36.8%) or remain essentially unaltered (tongue volume and volume of total soft tissues).[41]

CANDIDATE GENE APPROACHES

An initial strategy to evaluate gene variants conferring risk for OSA is to assess association with variants of candidate genes. There have been several candidate gene studies for OSA. Most of these studies have had very small sample sizes. Such small studies can have false-positive findings and need to be replicated in independent samples. Thus, all such studies are not described here. Rather, the author focuses on 2 polymorphisms that have been the most studied: apolipoprotein E ε4 (ApoE4) allele and a polymorphism of tumor necrosis factor α (TNF-α).

ApoE4

ApoE4 allele is a risk factor for Alzheimer disease.[43] For biological reasons that are a bit unclear, ApoE4 was also investigated as a risk factor for OSA. Both early positive associations[44] and negative[45] studies were reported. In the Sleep Heart Health Study, this association with OSA was found in younger subjects (younger than 65 years) but not in subjects older than 65 years.[46] But a recent meta-analysis combining data from 8 studies that allowed assessment of association of ApoE4 in 1901 cases and 4607 controls found no evidence of association.[47] Of the studies assessed, the strongest association was in a study in pediatric sleep apnea.[48]

Thus, there is no evidence that ApoE4 is a genetic risk factor for OSA. An alternative postulate as to the role of ApoE4 in OSA is that it might affect the consequences of the disorder.

Specifically, the question if patients with OSA with this allele show more cognitive impairment than others with similar degrees of OSA arises. In children, the association with ApoE4 and OSA is strongest in those with cognitive dysfunction.[48] In adults with OSA and the ApoE4 allele, there is more impairment of verbal memory than in other subjects with OSA.[49] Thus, there is some support for this assertion[50] but further studies are needed.

Polymorphisms of TNF-α

Another variant that has received some attention is within the TNF-α gene, that is, the TNF-α-308G polymorphism. This polymorphism is one of the several polymorphisms in the TNF-α, and TNF-α-308G is a variant in the promoter region. This particular allele increases promoter activity[51] and affects TNF-α production in vitro.[52,53] This polymorphism is associated with sleep apnea syndrome in adults, and siblings of patients with sleep apnea syndrome are significantly more likely to carry this allele.[54] When one compares the frequency of this polymorphism in obese patients with OSA to obese subjects without OSA there is a high prevalence of this polymorphism in the subjects with OSA (28.8% compared with 12.6% in those without OSA; $P = .001$).[55] One possibility to explain this association is that the presence of this polymorphism affects symptoms of OSA rather than being a risk factor for the disorder. Patients with symptoms are more likely to present clinically. It has been proposed that TNF-α levels may be an important determinant of sleepiness in disorders of excessive daytime sleepiness such as sleep apnea.[56,57] Moreover, administration of the TNF-α antagonist, etanercept, to sleepy patients with OSA reduces their sleepiness as measured by the multiple sleep latency test.[58] Thus, this TNF-α polymorphism may affect the degree of sleepiness in patients with OSA. This postulate is supported by recent data from studies of OSA in a pediatric population. Children with OSA who had the TNF-α polymorphism were more sleepy (mean Epworth Sleepiness Score $= 12.3 \pm 1.3$, [mean $\pm$ SD]) than those without the risk variant (mean Epworth Sleepiness Score $= 4.6 \pm 0.7$) and had higher TNF-α plasma levels (893.1 ± 34.8 vs 315.4 ± 17.8 pg/mL; $P<.0003$).[59] Whether this relationship between sleepiness in OSA and the TNF-α polymorphism occurs in adults is unknown and needs to be studied.

A BROAD CANDIDATE GENE STRATEGY

An alternative strategy is to evaluate the association with SNPs in a broad range of candidate genes from different pathways thought to be involved in the pathogenesis of OSA. This approach bears similarities to that proposed by Keating and colleagues[60] who developed a broad-based SNP chip for cardiovascular disease. In OSA, this approach has recently been reported by Larkin and colleagues.[61] The investigators identified the following potential pathways: craniofacial morphology (10 genes), obesity/inflammation (14 genes), ventilatory control (12 genes), and a pathway that was called pleiotropic/miscellaneous (16 genes). (The FTO gene described earlier was not included in the candidate list for obesity.) Larkin and colleagues identified tagged SNPs in these genes separately in whites of European origin (522 total tagged SNPs) and African Americans (1095 SNPs). The investigators looked separately in an African American sample and in a whites sample for association with OSA, both using AHI as a continuous variable, and for OSA defined as an AHI greater than or equal to 15 events per hour. Larkin and colleagues used a false discovery rate of 10% to define a positive association. There was no replication sample. Among the European Americans, 3 SNPs were associated with OSA as a dichotomous trait. The strongest association was with a SNP in the promoter region of the gene for the C-reactive protein (CRP). The other 2 SNPs were in the glial cell–derived neurotrophic factor gene (GDNF). In complementary analyses with AHI as a continuous trait, association with the same SNP in the CRP gene was found, as well as with 2 SNPs in the GDNF gene, albeit different SNPs than when assessed as a dichotomous trait.

A different pattern emerged in African Americans. An SNP in the serotonin 2A receptor was associated with OSA as a dichotomous trait at a false discovery rate less than 10%. No SNPs were associated with AHI as a continuous trait.

The investigators indicated the need to replicate these results. In recent in-silico analysis of white subjects with OSA who are part of the large Icelandic Sleep Apnea Cohort and who have been genotyped, these findings were not replicated.[62] No association was found between the reported SNPs in CRP or GDNF with moderate/severe OSA (ie, AHI$\geq$15 episodes per hour; 1425 patients and 24,981 controls) or with mild to moderate OSA (AHI$\geq$5 episodes per hour; 1711 patients and 24,981 controls) whether adjusted for BMI or not. None of the SNPs showed any effect on AHI in a quantitative trait locus analysis (P>.2 for all SNPs).

Thus, these findings have not been confirmed, and at present, without replication in other cohorts, it cannot be concluded that variants of CRP and GDNF in European Americans confer risk for OSA. The findings in African Americans

need to be validated in studies in this ethnic group. The makeup of the Icelandic population does not permit this analysis.

LINKAGE STUDIES

An alternative strategy is the assessment of genetic linkage. The only linkage studies reported to date all come from the Cleveland Family Study.[63–65] These studies have examined separately linkage in whites and African Americans. This strategy is based on the fact that different models were found for transmission of the genetic influence on OSA in European Americans and African Americans in their sample[18] (see discussion earlier). This strategy reduces the sample size available for linkage studies.

The initial linkage studies reported extremely modest linkage peaks for sleep apnea after controlling BMI as a covariate.[63,64] The logarithm of odds (LOD) scores were of the order of 1 (**Table 1**). These scores are not in the suggestive range for genome-wide significance. Previous standards for the interpretation of the LOD scores have been proposed to deal with false-positives.[66] An LOD score greater than 2.2 is considered suggestive and a score greater than 3.5 is considered genome-wide significant,[66] although some consider these cut points as being too conservative. The linkage approach used was to look for linkage with AHI across the lifespan in African Americans and whites. Both parents (average age in whites 72.6 years) and children (average age in whites 8 years) were included in the analysis.[63] These initial studies had very limited power; 63 probands in the study were whites with a total of 369 subjects.[63] In the study of African Americans, there were 54 probands and a total of 277 subjects.[64] The linkage peak found in African Americans was different from the 2 peaks found in whites (see **Table 1**).

Not surprisingly, a more recent study in the same cohort with a larger sample size failed to replicate any of these early findings.[65] Investigators indicated that this was likely because of lack of power in the early studies. In the more recent study, new linkage peaks with higher LOD scores were identified (see **Table 1**). These linkage peaks have not yet been replicated.

Somewhat surprisingly, in none of these reported linkage studies was fine mapping performed. With current genotyping technology, fine mapping is simple to perform. Fine mapping involves checking LOD scores for additional polymorphic markers in the linkage region identified. This serves to confirm the veracity of the linkage by replication, and narrow the region. Without fine mapping, it is

Table 1
Results of linkage studies

Ethnic Group	Chromosome Location	Unadjusted LOD Score	LOD Score After Adjustment for BMI
European Americans[63]	1p	1.39	No linkage
—	2p	1.64	1.33
—	12p	1.43	No linkage
—	1.40	1.45	—
European Americans[65]	6 (80.4 cM)	0.6	3.5
—	6 (182 cM)	4.7	0.4
—	10 (118.3 cM)	2.7	0.7
—	17 (74.6 cM)	0	1.9
African Americans[64]	8q24	1.29	1.09
African Americans[65]	8 (45 cM)	2.2	2.5
—	8 (100 cM)	1.31	0.4
—	8 (140 cM)	2.0	0.3
—	13 (49 cM)	2.0	0.3
—	18 (126 cM)	—	3.5
—	20 (telomeric end of p-arm)	3.9	2.2
—	22 (52 cM)	—	2.2

premature to discuss likely candidate genes. With linkage using around 400 polymorphic markers, there are several hundred genes between each marker.

It is conceivable that in OSA, which is likely to have substantial genetic heterogeneity and likely to be the result of gene variants in several pathways, linkage approaches will likely not identify genome-wide significant areas. Although linkage works well for mendelian disorders (single gene mutations with very large effect), it is a poor strategy to identify gene variants with modest effects.[67,68]

GWAS

As discussed in other articles in this issue by Schormair and Winklemann; and Faraco and Mignot, a powerful strategy to identify common gene variants with small effects is GWAS.[69] These studies involve comparing the frequency of a large number of SNPs between large numbers of patients and controls or looking for association with a quantitative trait. This approach, which was first successful in 2005 in macular degeneration,[70] is facilitated by genotyping platforms that simultaneously assess 500,000 to 1.0 million SNPs. Given the large number of genotype comparisons, this strategy design requires large numbers of subjects, statistical control for multiple comparisons, and a discovery phase with replication samples. Although only introduced in 2005, there have been more than 800 successful GWAS reported.[71] These include

studies on restless leg syndrome and narcolepsy that are reported in this issue (Schormair and Winkelmann and Faraco and Mignot, respectively). To date, there has been no report of a GWAS on OSA. A GWAS on OSA is a logical next step. It is likely that OSA is the result of many common genetic variants, each with small effects, and given this postulate, GWAS is a logical strategy. However, it may be that there will be necessity to reduce the degree of genetic heterogeneity in the sample by, for example, including only cases with a clear family history of OSA, as was done in the seminal study of genetics of restless legs syndrome[72] and/or choosing cases where the genetic pathway is likely to be similar, for example, using only relatively lean cases.

FUTURE

Given the complexity of sleep apnea with multiple known intermediate pathways with specific risk factors that are heritable, each will likely have many gene variants; consideration should be given to focusing on determining the gene variants for these different risk factors rather than for OSA, for example, of the known genes conferring risk for obesity, which, if any, are associated with OSA and are there gene variants that determine mandibular length. Although these gene variants may not be the most exciting and may not have the greatest clinical impact determining these variants makes it easier in the future to sort out other signals and determines truly interesting pathways that either confer risk for OSA or protect individuals who have the structural risk factors for the disorder but do not have apneas and hypopneas during sleep.

REFERENCES

1. Tregear S, Reston J, Schoelles K, et al. Continuous positive airway pressure reduces risk of motor vehicle crash among drivers with obstructive sleep apnea: systematic review and meta-analysis. Sleep 2010;33:1373–80.
2. Pack AI, Gislason T. Obstructive sleep apnea and cardiovascular disease: a perspective and future directions. Prog Cardiovasc Dis 2009;51:434–51.
3. Tasali E, Ip MS. Obstructive sleep apnea and metabolic syndrome: alterations in glucose metabolism and inflammation. Proc Am Thorac Soc 2008;5:207–17.
4. Hunter DJ, Kraft P. Drinking from the fire hose—statistical issues in genomewide association studies. N Engl J Med 2007;357:436–9.
5. Strohl KP, Saunders NA, Feldman NT, et al. Obstructive sleep apnea in family members. N Engl J Med 1978;299:969–73.
6. Redline S, Tosteson T, Tishler PV, et al. Studies in the genetics of obstructive sleep apnea. Familial aggregation of symptoms associated with sleep-related breathing disturbances. Am Rev Respir Dis 1992;145:440–4.
7. Redline S, Tishler PV, Tosteson TD, et al. The familial aggregation of obstructive sleep apnea. Am J Respir Crit Care Med 1995;151:682–7.
8. Guilleminault C, Partinen M, Hollman K, et al. Familial aggregates in obstructive sleep apnea syndrome. Chest 1995;107:1545–51.
9. Pillar G, Lavie P. Assessment of the role of inheritance in sleep apnea syndrome. Am J Respir Crit Care Med 1995;151:688–91.
10. Mathur R, Douglas NJ. Family studies in patients with the sleep apnea-hypopnea syndrome. Ann Intern Med 1995;122:174–8.
11. Gislason T, Johannsson JH, Haraldsson A, et al. Familial predisposition and cosegregation analysis of adult obstructive sleep apnea and the sudden infant death syndrome. Am J Respir Crit Care Med 2002;166:833–8.
12. Young T, Palta M, Dempsey J, et al. The occurrence of sleep-disordered breathing among middle-aged adults. N Engl J Med 1993;328:1230–5.
13. Stunkard AJ, Harris JR, Pedersen NL, et al. The body-mass index of twins who have been reared apart. N Engl J Med 1990;322:1483–7.
14. Comuzzie AG, Allison DB. The search for human obesity genes. Science 1998;280:1374–7.
15. Stunkard AJ, Foch TT, Hrubec Z. A twin study of human obesity. JAMA 1986;256:51–4.

16. Maes HH, Neale MC, Eaves LJ. Genetic and environmental factors in relative body weight and human adiposity. Behav Genet 1997;27:325–51.
17. Redline S, Tishler PV. The genetics of sleep apnea. Sleep Med Rev 2000;4:583–602.
18. Buxbaum SG, Elston RC, Tishler PV, et al. Genetics of the apnea hypopnea index in Caucasians and African Americans: I. Segregation analysis. Genet Epidemiol 2002;22:243–53.
19. Young T, Shahar E, Nieto FJ, et al. Predictors of sleep-disordered breathing in community-dwelling adults: the Sleep Heart Health Study. Arch Intern Med 2002;162:893–900.
20. Young T, Peppard PE, Gottlieb DJ. Epidemiology of obstructive sleep apnea: a population health perspective. Am J Respir Crit Care Med 2002;165:1217–39.
21. Patel SR, Larkin EK, Redline S. Shared genetic basis for obstructive sleep apnea and adiposity measures. Int J Obes (Lond) 2008;32:795–800.
22. Nashi N, Kang S, Barkdull GC, et al. Lingual fat at autopsy. Laryngoscope 2007;117:1467–73.
23. Brennick MJ, Pack AI, Ko K, et al. Altered upper airway and soft tissue structures in the New Zealand Obese mouse. Am J Respir Crit Care Med 2009;179:158–69.
24. Speliotes EK, Willer CJ, Berndt SI, et al. Association analyses of 249,796 individuals reveal 18 new loci associated with body mass index. Nat Genet 2010;42:937–48.
25. Tung YC, Yeo GS. From GWAS to biology: lessons from FTO. Ann N Y Acad Sci 2011;1220:162–71.
26. Tung YC, Ayuso E, Shan X, et al. Hypothalamic-specific manipulation of Fto, the ortholog of the human obesity gene FTO, affects food intake in rats. PLoS One 2010;5:e8771.
27. Gerken T, Girard CA, Tung YC, et al. The obesity-associated FTO gene encodes a 2-oxoglutarate-dependent nucleic acid demethylase. Science 2007;318:1469–72.
28. Miles PG, Vig PS, Weyant RJ, et al. Craniofacial structure and obstructive sleep apnea syndrome—a qualitative analysis and meta-analysis of the literature. Am J Orthod Dentofacial Orthop 1996;109:163–72.
29. Lowe AA, Fleetham JA, Adachi S, et al. Cephalometric and computed tomographic predictors of obstructive sleep apnea severity. Am J Orthod Dentofacial Orthop 1995;107:589–95.
30. Nelson S, Hans M. Contribution of craniofacial risk factors in increasing apneic activity among obese and nonobese habitual snorers. Chest 1997;111:154–62.
31. Okubo M, Suzuki M, Horiuchi A, et al. Morphologic analyses of mandible and upper airway soft tissue by MRI of patients with obstructive sleep apnea hypopnea syndrome. Sleep 2006;29:909–15.
32. Lee RW, Vasudavan S, Hui DS, et al. Differences in craniofacial structures and obesity in Caucasian

and Chinese patients with obstructive sleep apnea. Sleep 2010;33:1075–80.

33. Cakirer B, Hans MG, Graham G, et al. The relationship between craniofacial morphology and obstructive sleep apnea in whites and in African-Americans. Am J Respir Crit Care Med 2001;163:947–50.

34. Nance WE, Nakata M, Paul TD, et al. The use of twin studies in the analysis of phenotypic traits in man. In: Janerich TT, Skalko RG, Porter IH, editors. Congenital defects new directions in research. New York: Academic Press; 1974. p. 23–49.

35. Osborne RH, DeGeorge FV. Genetic basis of morphologic variation; an evaluation and application of the twin study method. Cambridge (MA): Harvard University Press; 1959.

36. Paoli JR, Lauwers F, Lacassagne L, et al. Craniofacial differences according to the body mass index of patients with obstructive sleep apnoea syndrome: cephalometric study in 85 patients. Br J Oral Maxillofac Surg 2001;39:40–5.

37. Sforza E, Bacon W, Weiss T, et al. Upper airway collapsibility and cephalometric variables in patients with obstructive sleep apnea. Am J Respir Crit Care Med 2000;161:347–52.

38. Tangugsorn V, Krogstad O, Espeland L, et al. Obstructive sleep apnoea: multiple comparisons of cephalometric variables of obese and non-obese patients. J Craniomaxillofac Surg 2000;28:204–12.

39. Chi L, Comyn F-L, Mitra N, et al. Identification of craniofacial risk factors for obstructive sleep apnea using three-dimensional MRI. Eur Respir J 2011. [Epub ahead of print].

40. Lee RW, Chan AS, Grunstein RR, et al. Craniofacial phenotyping in obstructive sleep apnea—a novel quantitative photographic approach. Sleep 2009;32:37–45.

41. Schwab RJ, Pasirstein M, Kaplan L, et al. Family aggregation of upper airway soft tissue structures in normal subjects and patients with sleep apnea. Am J Respir Crit Care Med 2006;173:453–63.

42. Schwab RJ, Pasirstein M, Pierson R, et al. Identification of upper airway anatomic risk factors for obstructive sleep apnea with volumetric magnetic resonance imaging. Am J Respir Crit Care Med 2003;168:522–30.

43. Bekris LM, Yu CE, Bird TD, et al. Genetics of Alzheimer disease. J Geriatr Psychiatry Neurol 2010;23:213–27.

44. Kadotani H, Kadotani T, Young T, et al. Association between apolipoprotein E epsilon4 and sleep-disordered breathing in adults. JAMA 2001;285:2888–90.

45. Foley DJ, Masaki K, White L, et al. Relationship between apolipoprotein E epsilon4 and sleep-disordered breathing at different ages. JAMA 2001;286:1447–8.

46. Gottlieb DJ, DeStefano AL, Foley DJ, et al. APOE epsilon4 is associated with obstructive sleep apnea/hypopnea: the Sleep Heart Health Study. Neurology 2004;63:664–8.

47. Thakre TP, Mamtani MR, Kulkarni H. Lack of association of the APOE epsilon 4 allele with the risk of obstructive sleep apnea: meta-analysis and meta-regression. Sleep 2009;32:1507–11.

48. Gozal D, Capdevila OS, Kheirandish-Gozal L, et al. APOE epsilon 4 allele, cognitive dysfunction, and obstructive sleep apnea in children. Neurology 2007;69:243–9.

49. Cosentino FI, Bosco P, Drago V, et al. The APOE epsilon4 allele increases the risk of impaired spatial working memory in obstructive sleep apnea. Sleep Med 2008;9:831–9.

50. Caselli RJ. Obstructive sleep apnea, apolipoprotein E e4, and mild cognitive impairment. Sleep Med 2008;9:816–7.

51. Kroeger KM, Carville KS, Abraham LJ. The -308 tumor necrosis factor-alpha promoter polymorphism effects transcription. Mol Immunol 1997;34:391–9.

52. Bouma G, Crusius JB, Oudkerk Pool M, et al. Secretion of tumour necrosis factor alpha and lymphotoxin alpha in relation to polymorphisms in the TNF genes and HLA-DR alleles. Relevance for inflammatory bowel disease. Scand J Immunol 1996;43:456–63.

53. Louis E, Franchimont D, Piron A, et al. Tumour necrosis factor (TNF) gene polymorphism influences TNF-alpha production in lipopolysaccharide (LPS)-stimulated whole blood cell culture in healthy humans. Clin Exp Immunol 1998;113:401–6.

54. Riha RL, Brander P, Vennelle M, et al. Tumour necrosis factor-alpha (-308) gene polymorphism in obstructive sleep apnoea-hypopnoea syndrome. Eur Respir J 2005;26:673–8.

55. Bhushan B, Guleria R, Misra A, et al. TNF-alpha gene polymorphism and TNF-alpha levels in obese Asian Indians with obstructive sleep apnea. Respir Med 2009;103:386–92.

56. Vgontzas AN, Papanicolaou DA, Bixler EO, et al. Elevation of plasma cytokines in disorders of excessive daytime sleepiness: role of sleep disturbance and obesity. J Clin Endocrinol Metab 1997;82:1313–6.

57. Vgontzas AN, Papanicolaou DA, Bixler EO, et al. Sleep apnea and daytime sleepiness and fatigue: relation to visceral obesity, insulin resistance, and hypercytokinemia. J Clin Endocrinol Metab 2000;85:1151–8.

58. Vgontzas AN, Zoumakis E, Lin HM, et al. Marked decrease in sleepiness in patients with sleep apnea by etanercept, a tumor necrosis factor-alpha antagonist. J Clin Endocrinol Metab 2004;89:4409–13.

59. Khalyfa A, Serpero LD, Kheirandish-Gozal L, et al. TNF-alpha gene polymorphisms and excessive daytime sleepiness in pediatric obstructive sleep apnea. J Pediatr 2011;158:77–82.

60. Keating BJ, Tischfield S, Murray SS, et al. Concept, design and implementation of a cardiovascular

gene-centric 50 k SNP array for large-scale genomic association studies. PLoS One 2008;3:e3583.

61. Larkin EK, Patel SR, Goodloe RJ, et al. A candidate gene study of obstructive sleep apnea in European-Americans and African-Americans. Am J Respir Crit Care Med 2010;182:947–53.

62. Gislason T, Pack A, Helgadottir H, et al. The CRP and GDNF genes do not contribute to apnea-hypopnea index or risk of obstructive sleep apnea [letter]. Am J Respir Crit Care Med, in press.

63. Palmer LJ, Buxbaum SG, Larkin E, et al. A whole-genome scan for obstructive sleep apnea and obesity. Am J Hum Genet 2003;72:340–50.

64. Palmer LJ, Buxbaum SG, Larkin EK, et al. Whole genome scan for obstructive sleep apnea and obesity in African-American families. Am J Respir Crit Care Med 2004;169:1314–21.

65. Larkin EK, Patel SR, Elston RC, et al. Using linkage analysis to identify quantitative trait loci for sleep apnea in relationship to body mass index. Ann Hum Genet 2008;72:762–73.

66. Lander E, Kruglyak L. Genetic dissection of complex traits: guidelines for interpreting and reporting linkage results. Nat Genet 1995;11:241–7.

67. Altmuller J, Palmer LJ, Fischer G, et al. Genomewide scans of complex human diseases: true linkage is hard to find. Am J Hum Genet 2001;69:936–50.

68. Risch NJ. Searching for genetic determinants in the new millennium. Nature 2000;405:847–56.

69. Hardy J, Singleton A. Genomewide association studies and human disease. N Engl J Med 2009;360:1759–68.

70. Edwards AO, Ritter R 3rd, Abel KJ, et al. Complement factor H polymorphism and age-related macular degeneration. Science 2005;308:421–4.

71. Hindorff LA, Junkins HA, Hall PN, et al. A catalog of published genome-wide association studies. Available at: www.genome.gov/gwastudies. Accessed May 12, 2011.

72. Winkelmann J, Schormair B, Lichtner P, et al. Genomewide association study of restless legs syndrome identifies common variants in three genomic regions. Nat Genet 2007;39:1000–6.

Genetics of Cardiovascular Consequences of Obstructive Sleep Apnea Syndrome

Silke Ryan, MD, PhD, Brian D. Kent, MB,
Walter T. McNicholas, MD*

KEYWORDS

- Obstructive sleep apnea syndrome
- Cardiovascular disease • Genetics • Obesity

Obstructive sleep apnea syndrome (OSAS) is a highly prevalent medical disorder affecting at least 4% of men and 2% of women in the developed world.[1] The disorder is characterized by repeated episodes of pharyngeal obstruction during sleep that lead to intermittent hypoxia, sleep fragmentation, and excessive daytime sleepiness.[2] OSAS is associated with significant morbidity and mortality. The excessive daytime sleepiness leads to impairments in quality of life, cognitive performance, and social functioning.[3] The major health burden in OSAS patients, however, is the strong risk of cardiovascular diseases, such as systemic arterial hypertension, coronary artery disease, heart failure, and stroke.[4] The association between OSAS and cardiovascular diseases has been suggested for many years, and more recently is corroborated by large-scale epidemiologic and prospective studies. The underlying mechanisms mediating this association are incompletely understood, but the pathogenesis is likely to be a multifactorial process.

In recent years, considerable effort has been made to understand the contribution of genetic factors to the development of OSAS involving genome-wide linkage studies and association studies of candidate genes. A detailed review on this subject is provided in an article by Pack and Gislason elsewhere in this issue. An increasing number of studies have also focused on the identification of a genetic basis for the cardiovascular pathogenesis in OSAS.

Following a brief summary of the current epidemiologic and clinical evidence of OSAS-associated cardiovascular involvement, this article provides a critical review on genetic factors that may contribute to the development of cardiovascular disorders in OSAS.

OSAS AND CARDIOVASCULAR DISEASES

An association between OSAS and the development of cardiovascular diseases has been suggested for several years. However, confounding variables such as obesity, hypertension, smoking, alcohol intake, age, and level of exercise made this independent relationship difficult to prove. Furthermore, many of the earlier studies on OSAS and cardiovascular diseases used samples from clinical populations, which are usually not representative of the condition in the general population and cannot be used to estimate the public health impact of the disease.[5] However, the

The authors have nothing to disclose.
Pulmonary and Sleep Disorders Unit, St. Vincent's University Hospital, Elm Park, Dublin 4, Ireland
* Corresponding author. Department of Respiratory Medicine, St. Vincent's University Hospital, Elm Park, Dublin 4, Ireland.
E-mail address: walter.mcnicholas@ucd.ie

Sleep Med Clin 6 (2011) 247–256
doi:10.1016/j.jsmc.2011.04.001

evidence of an association is growing, particularly with systemic arterial hypertension. Careful case-control studies have confirmed the association of OSAS and increased blood pressure independent of confounders such as obesity.[6] Also, data in patient and population samples extensively support a role for OSAS in the pathogenesis of hypertension.[7,8] In longitudinal population studies, OSAS increased the risk for increased blood pressure at follow-up.[9,10] The prevalence of OSAS is particularly high in patients with drug-resistant hypertension; a recent study found occult OSAS in up to 83% of patients who had uncontrolled hypertension despite taking 3 or more antihypertensive agents at optimum doses.[11] Data linking OSAS to other cardiovascular diseases are not as clear-cut, but nonetheless supportive. The strongest evidence is provided by data from the Sleep Heart Health Study cohort, which reports an independent association between OSAS and congestive cardiac failure, cerebrovascular disease, and coronary artery disease.[12] In support, Peker and colleagues[13] followed patients with known coronary artery disease for 5 years and observed a significantly higher mortality in patients with an apnea/hypopnea index (AHI; number of apneas and hypopneas per hour of sleep) of ≥10/h in comparison with matched controls.

Continuous positive airway pressure (CPAP) therapy, the most effective treatment for OSAS, decreases cardiovascular morbidity and mortality. Peker and colleagues[14] reported an increased incidence of cardiovascular disease among incompletely treated OSAS patients compared with those efficiently treated over a 7-year follow-up period. Furthermore, data from the authors' laboratory have demonstrated a reduction in deaths from cardiovascular causes in OSAS patients comparing CPAP-treated with untreated patients over an average follow-up of 7.5 years.[15] Similarly, in a large cardiovascular outcome study with a 10-year-period of follow-up, severe untreated OSAS significantly increased the risk of fatal and nonfatal cardiovascular events.[16]

The precise mechanisms of cardiovascular complications in OSAS have not yet been elucidated but are almost certainly of multiple etiology. The current concept of pathophysiology includes sympathetic excitation, endothelial dysfunction produced by inflammation and oxidative stress, increased coagulation, and metabolic dysregulation as possible mechanisms[4]; however, given the complexity of OSAS, a multifactorial pathogenesis is likely (**Fig. 1**). The unique form of hypoxia occurring in OSAS, with repetitive short cycles of desaturation followed by rapid reoxygenation, termed intermittent hypoxia (IH), along with sleep deprivation and sleep fragmentation, are likely the key mediators of the cardiovascular pathogenesis. With the growing knowledge of genetic factors contributing to the development of OSAS, there is also increasing interest in exploring a genetic contribution of the development of OSAS-related cardiovascular complications. In support of a potential genetic influence, Gami and colleagues[17] identified a significant and

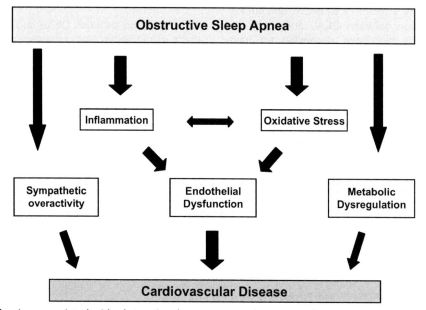

Fig. 1. Mechanisms associated with obstructive sleep apnea syndrome contributing to cardiovascular diseases.

independent association between OSAS and a familial history of mortality related to premature coronary artery disease.

GENETIC FACTORS OF CARDIOVASCULAR DISEASES IN OSAS
Systemic Inflammation

Accumulating evidence supports a central role for inflammation in all phases of atherosclerosis, from initiation of the fatty streak to the culmination in plaque rupture presenting as acute coronary syndrome.[18,19] Systemic inflammation occurs in the vasculature as a response to injury, lipid peroxidation, and perhaps infection.[20,21] Resident or circulating leukocytes mediate the adherence of monocytes to the endothelium, which in turn release several inflammatory mediators including cytokines such as tumor necrosis factor α (TNF-α) or interleukin (IL)-1, chemokines such as IL-8 or monocyte chemoattractant protein 1 (MCP-1), or adhesion molecules such as intercellular adhesion molecule 1 (ICAM-1) and selectins. Expression of adhesion molecules and chemokines facilitates the recruitment of macrophages, differentiated from monocytes, laden with oxidized lipid (foam cells). The accumulation of foam cells leads to the formation of a lipid pool, and production of collagen contributes to the strength of the fibrous cap. Cells also release IL-6, which is the main hepatic stimulus for the acute phase reactant, C-reactive protein (CRP), causing expression of adhesion molecules and mediating MCP-1 induction.[22]

There is growing evidence of activation of inflammatory pathways in OSAS.[23] IH is likely to play a significant role in the initiation of the inflammatory process through activation of the transcription factor nuclear factor κB (NF-κB).[24] This activation results in the expression of various proinflammatory cytokines such as TNF-α and IL-6, chemokines such as IL-8, adhesion molecules such as ICAM-1, and cell receptors. These mediators have also been linked to the pathogenesis of atherosclerosis and hypertension. Several studies have shown increased circulating levels of these markers in OSAS and a significant decrease with effective CPAP therapy.[25–31]

A genetic predisposition toward increased production of proinflammatory cytokine may contribute to this process. Riha and colleagues[32] demonstrated an independent association of the TNF-α (−308A) gene polymorphism with the diagnosis of OSAS in a Scottish population of 206 subjects. A similar association was found in an Indian population, and in this study the TNF-α (−308A) gene polymorphism was associated with an elevated circulating TNF-α level, supporting a potential

genetic predisposition for systemic inflammation in OSAS.[33] Moreover, a recent study detected an increased frequency of TNF-α (−308G) single nucleotide polymorphism (SNP) in a pediatric population with OSAS in comparison with matched controls, again associated with elevated circulating TNF-α levels; the investigators suggested that this phenomenon is related to excessive daytime sleepiness in this population.[34]

The role and significance of other inflammatory mediators are less clear. Earlier studies have suggested increased IL-6 levels in OSAS patients[30,31,35]; however, some of these reports may have been limited by smaller numbers, lack of adequately matched normal control populations, particularly in terms of body mass index (BMI), and the inclusion of patients with established cardiovascular or metabolic diseases. Recent studies did not detect an association between OSAS and IL-6.[27,36] A recent study by Zhang and colleagues[37] investigated the association of 5 IL-6 SNPs with OSAS and detected a linear increase of the AHI only in nonobese carriers of the C variant of IL-6 −572G/C polymorphism. This observation, however, was made in a small population and needs confirmation in larger studies.

Oxidative Stress

Oxidative stress occurs when there is an imbalance between the generation of reactive oxygen species (ROS) and antioxidants. Oxidative stress is associated with lipid and protein oxidation in the vascular wall, and is considered an early event in atherogenesis. However, as yet a specific causative relation between oxidative events in general and oxidative modification of low-density lipoprotein in particular with respect to atherosclerosis has not been determined, and clinical studies of the role of antioxidants have shown conflicting results.[38,39]

It has been proposed that the IH occurring in OSAS is analogous to ischemia-reperfusion injury, thus initiating oxidative stress and potentiating atherosclerotic sequelae in OSAS.[40,41] However, the issue of increased ROS production in OSAS is controversial. Two in vitro studies demonstrated increased ROS production from leukocytes of OSAS patients, which was reversed by CPAP therapy.[42,43] Several studies have also shown an increased intensity of lipid peroxidation that improved with CPAP therapy.[44–46] Furthermore, there is evidence of decreased antioxidant capacity as an indirect measure of enhanced oxidative stress in OSAS.[44,47] By contrast, Svatikova and colleagues[48] did not detect higher levels of lipid peroxidation biomarkers in exclusively normotensive OSAS patients in comparison with matched control subjects, and 2 further small studies failed to show increased oxidative stress in OSAS.[49,50]

Regarding a genetic basis for oxidative stress in OSAS, Lavie and colleagues[51] investigated the role of haptoglobin, which is a known antioxidant protein with immunomodulatory properties. Haptoglobin is encoded by two alleles with profoundly different biochemical and biophysical properties. This study included 465 subjects with OSAS and 757 controls, and a polymorphism in the haptoglobin gene was significantly associated with the presence of cardiovascular disease in younger patients. The reduced nicotinamide adenine dinucleotide phosphate (NADPH) oxidase complex is an important source of ROS. Liu and colleagues[52] assessed polymorphisms of the NADPH subunit p22phox in 176 Han Chinese persons, finding the T allele of the gene to be associated with AHI, nocturnal hypoxia, systolic blood pressure, and anthropometric measures of obesity. However, the association of this polymorphism with the development of cardiovascular disease was not investigated.

Endothelial Dysfunction

The endothelium is the major regulator of vascular homeostasis, maintaining vascular tone and controlling the equilibrium between inhibition and stimulation of smooth muscle cell proliferation, in addition to vascular thrombogenesis and fibrinolysis.[53,54] When this balance becomes upset endothelial dysfunction occurs, causing damage to the endothelial wall.[19] Endothelial dysfunction is considered an early marker for atherosclerosis.[55] The hallmark of endothelial dysfunction is impairment of endothelial-dependent vasodilatation, which is mediated by nitric oxide (NO). NO is the most potent vascular relaxing factor in the body and plays an important role as a signaling molecule in several biologic functions, including inflammation and neurotransmission. Various studies have demonstrated impairment in endothelium-mediated vasodilation by acetylcholine in OSAS, which acts through an NO-mediated pathway.[56,57] There is growing evidence of a critical role for NO in OSAS patients, and levels increase with CPAP therapy, suggesting that NO bioavailability is reduced in OSAS.[58,59] The association of eNOS4 and eNOS296 polymorphisms of the endothelial nitric oxide synthase (eNOS) gene with OSAS was investigated in a Turkish population of OSAS subjects and controls.[60] There was a significant difference between the patients and controls regarding eNOS296 polymorphism, but this was related to neither OSAS severity nor the presence of cardiovascular diseases. The endothelium also produces vasoconstrictor substances, such as endothelin-1. Studies on endothelin-1 concentrations in OSAS patients before and after CPAP therapy have produced conflicting results. Diefenbach and colleagues[61] evaluated the Lys198Asn endothelin-1 gene polymorphism and its relationship with OSAS in 364 patients and 57 healthy controls. Whereas they found no interaction between circulating endothelin-1 levels and the presence or severity of sleep-disordered breathing, the Lys198Asn variant was associated with more severe OSAS in obese persons. The same group also investigated polymorphisms of the endothelin receptor subtype A, finding that the G231A allele conferred a lower risk of OSAS, though with the caveat that this protective effect was observed in a relatively small control group.[62]

Angiotensin-Converting Enzyme Polymorphisms

The angiotensin-converting enzyme (ACE) plays an important role in blood pressure regulation and electrolyte balance by hydrolyzing angiotensin I into angiotensin II, a potent vasoconstrictor and aldosterone-stimulating peptide. The importance of this enzyme in the regulation of blood pressure is illustrated by the beneficial effect of ACE inhibitors in hypertension. An insertion/deletion (I/D, intron 16) polymorphism of the ACE gene correlates with circulating ACE plasma activity; higher plasma ACE activity is observed in subjects with ACE-D.[63,64] Several studies suggest an association between ACE-D and hypertension and cardiovascular disease,[65–67] therefore stimulating research on the importance of this polymorphism in the setting of OSAS.

In a Chinese population, Zhang and colleagues[68] found the ACE gene I/D polymorphism to be significantly associated with the severity of OSAS in a cohort of hypertensive subjects. In the Wisconsin Sleep Cohort including 1100 subjects, the I/D polymorphism was associated with hypertension, particularly in patients with mild to moderate OSAS.[69] Similar findings were obtained in a Brazilian male population.[70] Furthermore, the investigators suggested that the ACE I/I genotype may protect hypertensive men from developing severe OSAS. In direct contrast to the findings from the Wisconsin cohort, in participants enrolled in the Cleveland family study no significant association was found between ACE genotype and hypertension in subjects with mild to moderate OSAS but similarly, the ACE deletion allele seemed protective against hypertension in the setting of OSAS.[71] Two

Table 1
Candidate gene studies on cardiovascular aspects of obstructive sleep apnea syndrome

Gene	Allele	Finding	Population	References
TNF-α	−308 A/G	Association with OSAS but not hypertension	103 patients, 190 controls; Scotland	Riha et al[32]
	−308 A/G	Association with OSAS	104 patients, 103 controls; India	Bhushan et al[33]
Haptoglobin	1-1 2-1 2-2	2-2 polymorphism in OSAS patients <55 y associated with hypertension	465 OSAS patients, 757 controls; Israel	Lavie et al[51]
NADPH oxidase	P22phox subunit	T allele associated with AHI, BP, and BMI	107 patients, 69 controls; China	Liu et al[52]
eNOS	eNOS296	Predicts diagnosis of OSAS but not severity	48 patients, 181 controls; Turkey	Bayazit et al[60]
Endothelin-1	Lys198Asn	Associated with higher AHI in the obese	364 patients, 57 controls; Germany	Diefenbach et al[61]
ACE	I/D	Obesity related to D allele, uncertain association with OSAS and hypertension	174 subjects; China	Zhang et al[68]
	I/D	D allele associated with hypertension in mild-moderate OSAS	1100 subjects; Wisconsin Sleep Cohort	Lin et al[69]
	I/D	Hypertension risk reduced with D allele	972 subjects; Cleveland family study	Patel et al[71]
	I/D	Significant association of ACE polymorphism with OSAS and hypertension	157 patients with hypertension, 181 controls; Sweden	Bostrom et al[74]
β2-Adrenoreceptor	Cys47Arg Gly16Arg Gln27Glu	No significant association with BP, heart rate, lipid profile	429 patients with moderate to severe OSAS; Germany	Bartels et al[75]
ApoE	APOE4	No association between APOE4 and OSAS	1901 patients, 4607 controls; meta-analysis of 8 studies	Thakre et al[93]

Abbreviations: ACE, angiotensin-converting enzyme; AHI, apnea/hypopnea index; ApoE, apolipoprotein E; BMI, body mass index; BP, blood pressure; eNOS, endothelial nitric oxide synthase; I/D, insertion/deletion; NADPH, nicotinamide adenine dinucleotide phosphate; OSAS, obstructive sleep apnea syndrome; TNF-α, tumor necrosis factor α.

further studies failed to detect an association between ACE gene I/D polymorphism and hypertension in OSAS populations.[72,73] Applying a different approach, Bostrom and colleagues[74] studied a primary care cohort with newly diagnosed hypertension and matched controls. Sleep studies were performed to look for the presence of sleep-disordered breathing, which on interaction analysis was associated with ACE gene polymorphism and hypertension in men. However, the numbers in the study were small and confidence intervals high.

In summary, there is ongoing uncertainty regarding the association between ACE polymorphism and OSAS and its sequelae, and there is a clear need for larger, well-controlled studies.

Sympathetic Overactivity

Increased sympathetic neural activity is a hallmark of patients with OSAS, and likely plays a pivotal role in the development of comorbid hypertension. β-Adrenergic receptors mediate sympathetic activity and are regulators of lipid metabolism, insulin sensitivity, blood pressure, and heart rate. A limited number of studies in this area do not lend significant support to polymorphisms of these receptor genes driving the development of cardiovascular sequelae in OSAS.[75–77] Three β2-adrenergic polymorphisms (Cys47Arg, Gly16Arg, Gln27Glu) were examined in 429 German patients with moderate to severe OSAS, but no significant effect on blood pressure, heart rate, or lipid profile was detected.[75]

Obesity

Obesity is becoming a global epidemic, both in adults and children. Obesity and OSAS are intrinsically and intimately linked: the prevalence of OSAS in obese subjects exceeds 30%, and 60% to 90% of OSAS subjects are obese.[78] The incidence of OSAS increases sixfold for every 10 kg of weight gained in longitudinal studies.[79] Adipose tissue is metabolically active, and secretes humoral factors and adipokines that regulate the distribution of body fat.[80] Obesity and OSAS are often associated with dysregulation of glucose and lipid metabolism, and they share several associated comorbidities including cardiovascular disease, dyslipidemia, and diabetes mellitus, but the relative contribution of the two disorders to the development of these unwanted sequelae remains unclear. Visceral fat produces large amounts of proinflammatory cytokines that are thought to provoke inflammation, oxidative stress, cell adhesion, and endothelial dysfunction, and hence contribute to the development of atherosclerosis as well as the sleep-disordered breathing in association with the metabolic syndrome.[81]

The high prevalence of obesity in OSAS subjects has suggested a common genetic pathway. The most important studies performed exploring the interaction between OSAS and obesity have been based on the Cleveland family study, a longitudinal study consisting of individuals with OSAS, their family members, and neighborhood control families.[82] Palmer and colleagues[83] undertook a 9-cM genome scan in white pedigrees. Multipoint variance-component linkage analysis was performed for the OSA-associated quantitative phenotypes AHI and BMI. The investigators identified both shared and unshared genetic factors underlying susceptibility to OSAS and obesity, and concluded that there might be a common causal pathway. Similar conclusions were drawn from analysis of a genome-wide scan of an African American population; however, very different chromosome locations were found in comparison with the white population.[84] The significance of these findings is unknown (see the article by Pack and Gislason elsewhere in this issue).

Apolipoprotein E

Apolipoprotein E (ApoE) plays a major role in lipid metabolism. The expression of the ApoE4 isoform is considered to be a precursor of atherosclerosis, and is associated variably with the development of coronary artery disease as well as Alzheimer disease. Eight studies have examined the APOE4 genotype in the context of sleep-disordered breathing,[85–92] and the results have been recently summarized in a meta-analysis.[93] In the meta-analysis 6508 subjects were included, consisting of an OSAS population of 1901 cases and 4607 controls. There was a significant heterogeneity across the study results. Based on the results of the meta-analysis the investigators concluded that there is likely no association between ApoE polymorphisms and OSAS, but larger studies are needed before this hypothesis can definitely be refuted.

SUMMARY

OSAS is closely associated with many cardiovascular diseases. The pathogenesis of cardiovascular complications is OSAS is still incompletely understood, and the development of modern genetic investigative techniques has stimulated research into a potential genetic contribution to this association. Most studies investigated single candidate polymorphisms of various candidate genes (**Table 1**). As outlined in this article, studies so far have provided conflicting results, and numbers included have been small and consist of different populations, making comparisons between studies difficult. Furthermore, OSAS is a complex disorder consisting of various phenotypes. Therefore, the majority of cases of cardiovascular disease complicating OSAS are unlikely to be the product of distinct, focal gene polymorphisms. Many of the same problems apply to the study of essential hypertension and metabolic syndrome, making association studies more difficult.

Therefore, there is a clear need for large-scale multicenter studies of carefully defined patient and control populations using a combination of investigative methods. Such studies carry the prospect of evaluating potential genetic contributions to cardiovascular sequelae of OSAS, potentially unmasking certain target groups for specific intervention.

REFERENCES

1. Young T, Palta M, Dempsey J, et al. The occurrence of sleep-disordered breathing among middle-aged adults. N Engl J Med 1993;328:1230–5.
2. Guilleminault C, Tilkian A, Dement WC. The sleep apnea syndromes. Annu Rev Med 1976;27:465–84.
3. Engleman HM, Douglas NJ. Sleep. 4: sleepiness, cognitive function, and quality of life in obstructive sleep apnoea/hypopnoea syndrome. Thorax 2004; 59:618–22.
4. McNicholas WT, Bonsigore MR. Sleep apnoea as an independent risk factor for cardiovascular disease: current evidence, basic mechanisms and research priorities. Eur Respir J 2007;29:156–78.
5. Young T, Peppard PE, Gottlieb DJ. Epidemiology of obstructive sleep apnea: a population health perspective. Am J Respir Crit Care Med 2002;165: 1217–39.
6. Davies CW, Crosby JH, Mullins RL, et al. Case-control study of 24 hour ambulatory blood pressure in patients with obstructive sleep apnoea and normal matched control subjects. Thorax 2000;55: 736–40.
7. Nieto FJ, Young TB, Lind BK, et al. Association of sleep-disordered breathing, sleep apnea, and hypertension in a large community-based study. Sleep Heart Health Study. JAMA 2000;283:1829–36.
8. Young T, Peppard P, Palta M, et al. Population-based study of sleep-disordered breathing as a risk factor for hypertension. Arch Intern Med 1997;157: 1746–52.
9. Wright JT Jr, Redline S, Taylor AL, et al. Relationship between 24-h blood pressure and sleep disordered breathing in a normotensive community sample. Am J Hypertens 2001;14:743–8.
10. Peppard PE, Young T, Palta M, et al. Prospective study of the association between sleep-disordered breathing and hypertension. N Engl J Med 2000; 342:1378–84.
11. Logan AG, Perlikowski SM, Mente A, et al. High prevalence of unrecognized sleep apnoea in drug-resistant hypertension. J Hypertens 2001;19:2271–7.
12. Shahar E, Whitney CW, Redline S, et al. Sleep-disordered breathing and cardiovascular disease: cross-sectional results of the Sleep Heart Health Study. Am J Respir Crit Care Med 2001;163:19–25.
13. Peker Y, Hedner J, Kraiczi H, et al. Respiratory disturbance index: an independent predictor of mortality in coronary artery disease. Am J Respir Crit Care Med 2000;162:81–6.
14. Peker Y, Hedner J, Norum J, et al. Increased incidence of cardiovascular disease in middle-aged men with obstructive sleep apnea: a 7-year follow-up. Am J Respir Crit Care Med 2002;166:159–65.
15. Doherty LS, Kiely JL, Swan V, et al. Long-term effects of nasal continuous positive airway pressure therapy on cardiovascular outcomes in sleep apnea syndrome. Chest 2005;127:2076–84.
16. Marin JM, Carrizo SJ, Vicente E, et al. Long-term cardiovascular outcomes in men with obstructive sleep apnoea-hypopnoea with or without treatment with continuous positive airway pressure: an observational study. Lancet 2005;365:1046–53.
17. Gami AS, Rader S, Svatikova A, et al. Familial premature coronary artery disease mortality and obstructive sleep apnea. Chest 2007;131:118–21.
18. Libby P. Inflammation in atherosclerosis. Nature 2002;420:868–74.
19. Ross R. Atherosclerosis–an inflammatory disease. N Engl J Med 1999;340:115–26.
20. Glass CK, Witztum JL. Atherosclerosis. the road ahead. Cell 2001;104:503–16.
21. Lusis AJ. Atherosclerosis. Nature 2000;407:233–41.
22. Pasceri V, Willerson JT, Yeh ET. Direct proinflammatory effect of C-reactive protein on human endothelial cells. Circulation 2000;102:2165–8.
23. Ryan S, Taylor CT, McNicholas WT. Systemic inflammation: a key factor in the pathogenesis of cardiovascular complications in obstructive sleep apnoea syndrome? Thorax 2009;64:631–6.
24. Ryan S, Taylor CT, McNicholas WT. Selective activation of inflammatory pathways by intermittent hypoxia in obstructive sleep apnea syndrome. Circulation 2005;112:2660–7.
25. Dyugovskaya L, Lavie P, Lavie L. Phenotypic and functional characterization of blood gammadelta T cells in sleep apnea. Am J Respir Crit Care Med 2003;168:242–9.
26. Minoguchi K, Tazaki T, Yokoe T, et al. Elevated production of tumor necrosis factor-alpha by monocytes in patients with obstructive sleep apnea syndrome. Chest 2004;126:1473–9.

27. Ryan S, Taylor CT, McNicholas WT. Predictors of elevated nuclear factor-kappaB-dependent genes in obstructive sleep apnea syndrome. Am J Respir Crit Care Med 2006;174:824–30.

28. Ohga E, Tomita T, Wada H, et al. Effects of obstructive sleep apnea on circulating ICAM-1, IL-8, and MCP-1. J Appl Physiol 2003;94:179–84.

29. Ursavas A, Karadag M, Rodoplu E, et al. Circulating ICAM-1 and VCAM-1 levels in patients with obstructive sleep apnea syndrome. Respiration 2007;74: 525–32.

30. Vgontzas AN, Papanicolaou DA, Bixler EO, et al. Elevation of plasma cytokines in disorders of excessive daytime sleepiness: role of sleep disturbance and obesity. J Clin Endocrinol Metab 1997;82:1313–6.

31. Yokoe T, Minoguchi K, Matsuo H, et al. Elevated levels of C-reactive protein and interleukin-6 in patients with obstructive sleep apnea syndrome are decreased by nasal continuous positive airway pressure. Circulation 2003;107:1129–34.

32. Riha RL, Brander P, Vennelle M, et al. Tumour necrosis factor-alpha (-308) gene polymorphism in obstructive sleep apnoea-hypopnoea syndrome. Eur Respir J 2005;26:673–8.

33. Bhushan B, Guleria R, Misra A, et al. TNF-alpha gene polymorphism and TNF-alpha levels in obese Asian Indians with obstructive sleep apnea. Respir Med 2009;103:386–92.

34. Khalyfa A, Serpero LD, Kheirandish-Gozal L, et al. TNF-alpha gene polymorphisms and excessive daytime sleepiness in pediatric obstructive sleep apnea. J Pediatr 2011;158(1):77–82.

35. Ciftci TU, Kokturk O, Bukan N, et al. The relationship between serum cytokine levels with obesity and obstructive sleep apnea syndrome. Cytokine 2004; 28:87–91.

36. Mehra R, Storfer-Isser A, Kirchner HL, et al. Soluble interleukin 6 receptor: A novel marker of moderate to severe sleep-related breathing disorder. Arch Intern Med 2006;166:1725–31.

37. Zhang X, Liu RY, Lei Z, et al. Genetic variants in interleukin-6 modified risk of obstructive sleep apnea syndrome. Int J Mol Med 2009;23:485–93.

38. Lefer DJ, Granger DN. Oxidative stress and cardiac disease. Am J Med 2000;109:315–23.

39. Molavi B, Mehta JL. Oxidative stress in cardiovascular disease: molecular basis of its deleterious effects, its detection, and therapeutic considerations. Curr Opin Cardiol 2004;19:488–93.

40. Dean RT, Wilcox I. Possible atherogenic effects of hypoxia during obstructive sleep apnea. Sleep 1993;16:S15–21 [discussion: S21–12].

41. Lavie L. Obstructive sleep apnoea syndrome—an oxidative stress disorder. Sleep Med Rev 2003;7: 35–51.

42. Dyugovskaya L, Lavie P, Lavie L. Increased adhesion molecules expression and production of reactive oxygen species in leukocytes of sleep apnea patients. Am J Respir Crit Care Med 2002; 165:934–9.

43. Schulz R, Mahmoudi S, Hattar K, et al. Enhanced release of superoxide from polymorphonuclear neutrophils in obstructive sleep apnea. Impact of continuous positive airway pressure therapy. Am J Respir Crit Care Med 2000;162:566–70.

44. Barcelo A, Barbe F, de la Pena M, et al. Antioxidant status in patients with sleep apnoea and impact of continuous positive airway pressure treatment. Eur Respir J 2006;27:756–60.

45. Barcelo A, Miralles C, Barbe F, et al. Abnormal lipid peroxidation in patients with sleep apnoea. Eur Respir J 2000;16:644–7.

46. Lavie L, Vishnevsky A, Lavie P. Evidence for lipid peroxidation in obstructive sleep apnea. Sleep 2004;27:123–8.

47. Christou K, Moulas AN, Pastaka C, et al. Antioxidant capacity in obstructive sleep apnea patients. Sleep Med 2003;4:225–8.

48. Svatikova A, Wolk R, Lerman LO, et al. Oxidative stress in obstructive sleep apnoea. Eur Heart J 2005;26:2435–9.

49. Ozturk L, Mansour B, Yuksel M, et al. Lipid peroxidation and osmotic fragility of red blood cells in sleep-apnea patients. Clin Chim Acta 2003;332:83–8.

50. Wali SO, Bahammam AS, Massaeli H, et al. Susceptibility of LDL to oxidative stress in obstructive sleep apnea. Sleep 1998;21:290–6.

51. Lavie L, Lotan R, Hochberg I, et al. Haptoglobin polymorphism is a risk factor for cardiovascular disease in patients with obstructive sleep apnea syndrome. Sleep 2003;26:592–5.

52. Liu HG, Liu K, Zhou YN, et al. Relationship between reduced nicotinamide adenine dinucleotide phosphate oxidase subunit p22phox gene polymorphism and obstructive sleep apnea-hypopnea syndrome in the Chinese Han population. Chin Med J (Engl) 2009;122:1369–74.

53. Kinlay S, Libby P, Ganz P. Endothelial function and coronary artery disease. Curr Opin Lipidol 2001; 12:383–9.

54. Trepels T, Zeiher AM, Fichtlscherer S. The endothelium and inflammation. Endothelium 2006;13: 423–9.

55. Schachinger V, Britten MB, Zeiher AM. Prognostic impact of coronary vasodilator dysfunction on adverse long-term outcome of coronary heart disease. Circulation 2000;101:1899–906.

56. Kato M, Roberts-Thomson P, Phillips BG, et al. Impairment of endothelium-dependent vasodilation of resistance vessels in patients with obstructive sleep apnea. Circulation 2000;102:2607–10.

57. Kraiczi H, Hedner J, Peker Y, et al. Increased vasoconstrictor sensitivity in obstructive sleep apnea. J Appl Physiol 2000;89:493–8.

58. Ip MS, Lam B, Chan LY, et al. Circulating nitric oxide is suppressed in obstructive sleep apnea and is reversed by nasal continuous positive airway pressure. Am J Respir Crit Care Med 2000;162:2166–71.

59. Schulz R, Schmidt D, Blum A, et al. Decreased plasma levels of nitric oxide derivatives in obstructive sleep apnoea: response to CPAP therapy. Thorax 2000;55:1046–51.

60. Bayazit YA, Yilmaz M, Erdal E, et al. Role of nitric oxide synthase gene intron 4 and exon 7 polymorphisms in obstructive sleep apnea syndrome. Eur Arch Otorhinolaryngol 2009;266:449–54.

61. Diefenbach K, Kretschmer K, Bauer S, et al. Endothelin-1 gene variant Lys198Asn and plasma endothelin level in obstructive sleep apnea. Cardiology 2009;112:62–8.

62. Buck D, Diefenbach K, Penzel T, et al. Genetic polymorphisms in endothelin-receptor-subtype-a-gene as susceptibility factor for obstructive sleep apnea syndrome. Sleep Med 2010;11:213–7.

63. Agerholm-Larsen B, Nordestgaard BG, Tybjaerg-Hansen A. ACE gene polymorphism in cardiovascular disease: meta-analyses of small and large studies in whites. Arterioscler Thromb Vasc Biol 2000;20:484–92.

64. Rigat B, Hubert C, Alhenc-Gelas F, et al. An insertion/deletion polymorphism in the angiotensin I-converting enzyme gene accounting for half the variance of serum enzyme levels. J Clin Invest 1990;86:1343–6.

65. Danser AH, Schalekamp MA, Bax WA, et al. Angiotensin-converting enzyme in the human heart. Effect of the deletion/insertion polymorphism. Circulation 1995;92:1387–8.

66. O'Donnell CJ, Lindpaintner K, Larson MG, et al. Evidence for association and genetic linkage of the angiotensin-converting enzyme locus with hypertension and blood pressure in men but not women in the Framingham Heart Study. Circulation 1998;97:1766–72.

67. Schunkert H, Hense HW, Holmer SR, et al. Association between a deletion polymorphism of the angiotensin-converting-enzyme gene and left ventricular hypertrophy. N Engl J Med 1994;330:1634–8.

68. Zhang J, Zhao B, Gesongluobu, et al. Angiotensin-converting enzyme gene insertion/deletion (I/D) polymorphism in hypertensive patients with different degrees of obstructive sleep apnea. Hypertens Res 2000;23:407–11.

69. Lin L, Finn L, Zhang J, et al. Angiotensin-converting enzyme, sleep-disordered breathing, and hypertension. Am J Respir Crit Care Med 2004;170:1349–53.

70. Koyama RG, Drager LF, Lorenzi-Filho G, et al. Reciprocal interactions of obstructive sleep apnea and hypertension associated with ACE I/D polymorphism in males. Sleep Med 2009;10:1107–11.

71. Patel SR, Larkin EK, Mignot E, et al. The association of angiotensin converting enzyme (ACE) polymorphisms with sleep apnea and hypertension. Sleep 2007;30:531–3.

72. Barcelo A, Elorza MA, Barbe F, et al. Angiotensin converting enzyme in patients with sleep apnoea syndrome: plasma activity and gene polymorphisms. Eur Respir J 2001;17:728–32.

73. Yakut T, Karkucak M, Ursavas A, et al. Lack of association of ACE gene I/D polymorphism with obstructive sleep apnea syndrome in Turkish patients. Genet Mol Res 2010;9:734–8.

74. Bostrom KB, Hedner J, Melander O, et al. Interaction between the angiotensin-converting enzyme gene insertion/deletion polymorphism and obstructive sleep apnoea as a mechanism for hypertension. J Hypertens 2007;25:779–83.

75. Bartels NK, Borgel J, Wieczorek S, et al. Risk factors and myocardial infarction in patients with obstructive sleep apnea: impact of beta2-adrenergic receptor polymorphisms. BMC Med 2007;5:1.

76. Borgel J, Schulz T, Bartels NK, et al. Modifying effects of the R389G beta1-adrenoceptor polymorphism on resting heart rate and blood pressure in patients with obstructive sleep apnoea. Clin Sci (Lond) 2006;110:117–23.

77. Pierola J, Barcelo A, de la Pena M, et al. beta3-Adrenergic receptor Trp64Arg polymorphism and increased body mass index in sleep apnoea. Eur Respir J 2007;30:743–7.

78. Gami AS, Caples SM, Somers VK. Obesity and obstructive sleep apnea. Endocrinol Metab Clin North Am 2003;32:869–94.

79. Peppard PE, Young T, Palta M, et al. Longitudinal study of moderate weight change and sleep-disordered breathing. JAMA 2000;284:3015–21.

80. de Sousa AG, Cercato C, Mancini MC, et al. Obesity and obstructive sleep apnea-hypopnea syndrome. Obes Rev 2008;9:340–54.

81. Pillar G, Shehadeh N. Abdominal fat and sleep apnea: the chicken or the egg? Diabetes Care 2008;31(Suppl 2):S303–9.

82. Redline S, Tishler PV, Tosteson TD, et al. The familial aggregation of obstructive sleep apnea. Am J Respir Crit Care Med 1995;151:682–7.

83. Palmer LJ, Buxbaum SG, Larkin E, et al. A whole-genome scan for obstructive sleep apnea and obesity. Am J Hum Genet 2003;72:340–50.

84. Palmer LJ, Buxbaum SG, Larkin EK, et al. Whole genome scan for obstructive sleep apnea and obesity in African-American families. Am J Respir Crit Care Med 2004;169:1314–21.

85. Cosentino FI, Bosco P, Drago V, et al. The APOE epsilon4 allele increases the risk of impaired spatial working memory in obstructive sleep apnea. Sleep Med 2008;9:831–9.

86. Craig D, Hart DJ, Passmore AP. Genetically increased risk of sleep disruption in Alzheimer's disease. Sleep 2006;29:1003–7.

87. Foley DJ, Masaki K, White L, et al. Relationship between apolipoprotein E epsilon4 and sleep-disordered breathing at different ages. JAMA 2001;286:1447–8.

88. Gottlieb DJ, DeStefano AL, Foley DJ, et al. APOE epsilon4 is associated with obstructive sleep apnea/hypopnea: the Sleep Heart Health Study. Neurology 2004;63:664–8.

89. Gozal D, Capdevila OS, Kheirandish-Gozal L, et al. APOE epsilon 4 allele, cognitive dysfunction, and obstructive sleep apnea in children. Neurology 2007;69:243–9.

90. Kadotani H, Kadotani T, Young T, et al. Association between apolipoprotein E epsilon4 and sleep-disordered breathing in adults. JAMA 2001;285: 2888–90.

91. Larkin EK, Patel SR, Redline S, et al. Apolipoprotein E and obstructive sleep apnea: evaluating whether a candidate gene explains a linkage peak. Genet Epidemiol 2006;30:101–10.

92. Saarelainen S, Lehtimaki T, Kallonen E, et al. No relation between apolipoprotein E alleles and obstructive sleep apnea. Clin Genet 1998;53:147–8.

93. Thakre TP, Mamtani MR, Kulkarni H. Lack of association of the APOE epsilon 4 allele with the risk of obstructive sleep apnea: meta-analysis and meta-regression. Sleep 2009;32:1507–11.

Index

Note: Page numbers of article titles are in **boldface** type.

A

Adenosine, genes that affect neurotransmission by, relationship to insomnia, 197

Adenosine-related polymorphisms, candidate gene studies of sleep deprivation, 178

Angiotensin-converting enzyme polymorphisms, genetics of, in obstructive sleep apnea syndrome, 250–252

Animal models, genetic of sleep in rodent models, **141–154**
    genetic studies of electroencephalography in, 160–163
    non-mammalian genetic model systems in sleep research, **131–139**
    of narcolepsy, 221–222

Apnea. See Obstructive sleep apnea.

APoE4, in obstructive sleep apnea, 240

Apolipoprotein E, genetics of, in obstructive sleep apnea syndrome, 252

Arousal, from NREM sleep, genetics of disorders of, 229–231
    confusional arousals, 230
    sleep terrors, 230–231
    sleepwalking, 230

Association studies, of restless legs syndrome, 208–211
    candidate genes, 208–210
    genome-wide, 210–211
    in RLS linkage regions, 211

Autoimmunity, human leukocyte antigen (HLA) association in narcolepsy, 221

C

Caenorhabditis elegans (C elegans), genetic models systems in sleep research in, **131–139**

Candidate gene studies, association studies in restless legs syndrome, 208–210
    in obstructive sleep apnea, 240–241
        APoE4, 240
        broad strategy for, 240–241
        polymorphisms of TNF-α, 240
    of genes related to insomnia, 195–197
        adenosine, 197
        dopamine, 196–197
        gamma-aminobutyric acid, 197
        hypocretin/orexin, 197
        serotonin, 196

Cardiovascular disease, genetics of cardiovascular consequences of obstructive sleep apnea, **247–256**
    association between, 247–249
    genetic factors in, 249–252
        angiotensin-converting enzyme polymorphisms, 250–252
        apolipoprotein E, 252
        endothelial dysfunction, 250
        obesity, 252
        oxidative stress, 249–250
        sympathetic overactivity, 252
        systemic inflammation, 249

Catechol-O-methyltransferase (COMT) Val158Met polymorphism, candidate gene studies of sleep deprivation, 178

Chronic disease, genetics of, link to genetics of sleep, 150–151

Circadian rhythm disorders, genetics of disorders of, **183–190**
    diagnosis and prevalence, 186
    genetic basis of sleep disorders of, 188
    pathophysiology, 186–187

Circadian rhythms, disruption in rodent models, alterations in sleep due to, 148–150
    in mammals, 183–184
    in non-mammalian genetic model systems in sleep research on, 131–133
    individual differences in timing of sleep and, 172–173

Confusional arousals, genetics of, 230

Craniofacial structure, intermediate trait for obstructive sleep apnea, 239

D

Dissociative disorders, sleep-related, genetics of, 233

Dopamine transporter gene, related to insomnia, 196–197

DQB1*0602 allele, in candidate gene studies of sleep deprivation, 174–178

Drosophila, genetic models systems in sleep research in, **131–139**

Duration, sleep, genetics of, **171–182**

E

Eating disorders, sleep-related, genetics of, 234

Electroencephalography, genetics of, during wakefulness and sleep, **155–169**

doi:10.1016/S1556-407X(11)00050-6

Printed and bound by CPI Group (UK) Ltd, Croydon, CR0 4YY

03/10/2024

01040355-0018